Essential Cardiac Technology

FOR THE STUDENT HEALTH CARE PROFESSIONAL

Laurence W. Piller

Cardiac Clinic, Department of Medicine,
University of Cape Town and Groote Schuur Hospital,
South Africa

ho
ap

harwood academic publishers

Australia • China • France • Germany • India • Japan • Luxembourg
Malaysia • Russia • Singapore • Switzerland • Thailand • The Netherlands
United Kingdom • United States

3 Boulevard Royal
L-2449 Luxembourg

British Library Cataloguing in Publication Data
Pending

ISBN 3-7186-5897-6 (SC)
ISBN 3-7186-5896-8 (HC)

Printed and bound by The Rustica Press (Pty) Ltd, Old Mill Road, Ndabeni

Rustica—D4345

To my son Richard and
in loving memory of my daughter Linda Jane

Acknowledgments

I gratefully acknowledge the encouragement of many of my clinical technologist colleagues, both students and registered, without which this work would never have been completed. To my friends, Lydia Beckman, Helen Clark and Gary Mead, my thanks for their contributions. My thanks also to Mladin Polluta of the Department of Bio-Engineering, University of Cape Town, who gave precious time in providing valued comments. I am also most grateful to Dirk Kotze for his expert editing assistance.

I owe special thanks for the support given by Professor SR Benatar, head of the Department of Medicine, University of Cape Town, and to Professor PJ Commerford, director of Cardiology, Groote Schuur Hospital, both for valuable assistance and for access to the Medical Graphics Department. I am indebted to Ms. Pat Carstens for her generous and enduring secretarial help.

Foreword

It is now 30 years since Laurence Piller published his book *Manual of Cardio-Pulmonary Technology*. Although written primarily for the cardiac technologist, it proved to be a valuable resource for a generation of cardiology registrars, including myself, and for other professionals involved in cardiovascular care. It provided a clear and concise introduction to the complexities of cardiac technology during the formative years of this speciality.

This new book is a worthy successor to the original publication. The current management of the patient with cardiovascular disease involves the utilization of an increasing array of complex technological innovations. This book succeeds admirably in providing an understanding of the new developments and techniques of the past ten to twenty years used to diagnose and treat cardiovascular disease.

It is a particular pleasure for me to write this foreword in a book written by Mr Piller, who after training at the National Heart Hospital in London, England, emigrated to South Africa. He has held the position of Chief Technologist in cardiology at Groote Schuur Hospital in Cape Town for the past 25 years. He is a Fellow of the Society of Clinical technologists (Cardiology) in both South Africa and the United Kingdom; a member of the American Society of Cardiovascular Professionals and the author of many publications dealing with technical cardiology. These facts, however, do not do justice to the role that Mr Piller, or Bill as he is known to most of us, has played in the development of cardiology in South Africa. He was a key member of the Cardiac Clinic at Groote Schuur Hospital under Professor V Schrire at a time when the foundations of excellence in cardiology and cardiac surgery were becoming firmly established.

This is an excellent book that reflects the expertise and teaching skills of the author and I am certain that it will be useful to all who are directly involved in clinical cardiac technology, including technologists, nurses, radiographers and their physician colleagues, and also those who may have indirect involvement, such as bio-engineers, clinical engineers and technical staff of manufacturing and distribution companies.

BERNARD J GERSH, MB, CHB, DPHIL, FRCP
Teaching Professor of Cardiology; Chief, Division of Cardiology, Georgetown University Medical Center, Washington DC. USA

Preface

During the past decade cardiac technology has advanced at a greater pace than at any other period during the past sixty years, and almost every aspect of the profession has created its own subject speciality. The technologist and nurse employed in a busy cardiology centre may be classified as Invasive or Non-invasive and/or further sub-classified as Cath Lab, Echo, EP or ICU, each demanding specific knowledge and expertise. In writing this book I have attempted to explain the fundamentals of most of the common instrumentation techniques that are presently in use in many cardiac centres for the diagnoses and treatments of heart disease. It is acknowledged that not all institutions are fortunate to possess the advanced and very expensive equipment that is available. For this reason I have made mention of some less up-to-date technology, and accept that changes and new methods of diagnosis and treatment of heart disease will take place, even during the publication of this work.

The reader who desires further information is advised to consult some of the many excellent publications available. It is, however, hoped that the contents will "whet the appetite" of the student and also be of some value to his/her medical colleagues who are employed in cardiology or related fields.

LW PILLER
Cape Town, 1995

Contents

1 *Electrocardiography*

For more than one hundred years scientists, physicians and, in more recent years, electrophysiologists have studied the human electrocardiogram. It is a subject that today is still without absolute reason and understanding. It is well to diagnose an electrocardiographic abnormality by a change of its pattern from normality. It is another matter to understood the reason and cause of that change. Let us first be aware that to understand the fundamentals of electrocardiography it is necessary for the student to consider two important facts:

(a) The electrical potentials generated by the heart and recorded as an electrocardiographic waveform are, in effect, the sum of the *resultant potentials* of each of the individual myocardial cells, and the shape or morphology of the recorded event is dependent upon the direction in which the electrical forces are propagated.

(b) The electrocardiogram is an alternating current (AC) signal of a few millivolts amplitude that is superimposed upon a static direct current (DC) signal within the range of a few milli-volts to a few hundred in amplitude. When recorded, this D.C. voltage on which the ECG is superimposed may be either blocked by an electrical capacitor in the input circuit of the ECG machine, allowing only the alternating component of the ECG to be recorded in which case the low frequency response of the machine would be 0.05 Hz or alternatively, and today more frequently, blocked by a direct current restoring circuit that gives a *low frequency response* of zero Hz.

THE ACTION POTENTIAL

Perhaps a resumé of how the cells of the heart generate electrical potentials should be discussed at this point.

Each of the cardiac cells consists of a membrane which contains a nucleus surrounded by a substance known as cytoplasm. This membrane allows nutrients to pass into the cell and waste products to escape from it. Non-beneficial substances are excluded from entering, thereby retaining the composition of the cell. This unique property, known as *selective permeability* avoids the infiltration of sodium ions (Na+) into the cell; at the same time preventing potassium ions (K+) from leaving the cell. By the process of *osmosis* (which allows fluid to diffuse through a permeable membrane from a more to a less dense medium) certain substances e.g. oxygen, water, carbon dioxide, glucose, electrolytic ions, etc., readily difuse through the membrane, whilst others e.g. proteins, enzymes, hormones, some electrolytic ions, amino acids, etc., will not be accepted unless they are actively transported.

This mechanism of *active transportation* also allows certain substances to diffuse in the opposite direction, i.e. from a lesser dense medium to a higher dense medium.

Related to nerve and muscle cells of the heart we are mainly concerned with two of these substances, viz. Sodium (Na+), contained outside the cell membrane, and Potassium (K+), contained in abundance within the cell. When potassium molecules diffuse through the membrane to the outside they are returned by active transport mechanisms to within the cell. One must assume that similar mechanisms will return any sodium molecules should they enter the cell. This transport of Na+ and K+ from within and without the cell is known as the *sodium pump* of the cell and plays an important part in nerve and muscle action.

Another important consideration is the existence of a *potential difference* across the membrane of all cells, including the cardiac myocyte and *Purkinje cells*, of approximately 90 mV during the resting phase, known as the *resting membrane potential*. The inside of the cell negatively charged with respect to its extracellular environment.

It is the function of the cell to maintain the normal ratio of charge of ions across the cell membrane. In doing so each cell expends an enormous amount of energy in active transport of the various substances and, in order that the cell may respond to a stimulus, it must of necessity produce a change in its resting membrane potential. When the cell is resting it is in a state of *polarisation* or said to be `polarised'. In other words there exists the normal level of sodium ions outside the cell and the normal amount of potassium ions plus large organic negative ions within the cell.

Should, however, the cell receive a stimulus of any kind, such as mechanical, electrical, or chemical, it will immediately allow the membrane to become permeable to the sodium ions until the entire cell is invaded. This invasion of sodium ions causes the cell to contain more positive than negative ions and momentarily reverses the membrane potential to approximately +20 mV. This process of *depolarisation* causes the protein components of the cell, known as *myofibrils*, to shorten. The effect is contraction of the cell.

The uniqueness of the cardiac cell allows it to retain its positivity much longer than other cells in the body and thereby lengthening the contraction time to around 300 milliseconds. During this period of depolarisation, and as long as the cell is electrically positive, it cannot again be stimulated. This is termed the *absolute refractory period* and is particularly long in the myocardial cell, some 250 ms.

FIGURE 1

Myocardial Refractory
Periods. AR — Absolute
Refractory,
RR — Relative
Refractory

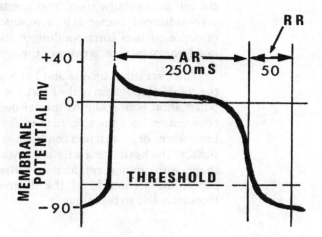

Once the myofibrils have shortened, *repolarisation* takes place as the sodium ions quickly diffuse from the cell, allowing it to revert to its original state. However as the resting membrane potential approaches its normal level there is a period when the cell may accept a further stimulation, but only if of sufficient strength. This period of refractoriness is known as the *relative refractory period* of some 50 ms duration in the myocardial cell. The total refractory period i.e. absolute plus relative, ensures that there can be no extension of the depolarisation wave once it has traversed its normal pathway.

When repolarisation is almost complete there is a very short period, known as the *supernormal phase*, and it is at this time that the cell may be hyperexcitable and, if stimulated, respond abnormally. This period of hypersensitivity is often pronounced in the presence of ischemic heart disease and is believed to be responsible for the associated high incidence of arrhythmias in patients with this condition. It coincides with the so-called *vulnerable zone* of the electrocardiogram.

Another uniqueness of cardiac cells is that they are in electrical communication with each other. Excitation of one cell will cause adjacent cells to respond. Some cells, e.g. those of the His bundle and its branches and the conduction tracts within the atrium are able to transmit impulses very rapidly whilst those of the AV node transmit at a much slower rate. This slowing of conduction through the AV node allows time for the ventricles to be filled with blood from the atria prior to ejection of their contents into the major arteries. Cells of the SA node on the other hand leak sodium at a relatively slow rate until the cell membrane breaks down causing the cell to depolarise itself. This special electrical property of the myocardial cell, known as its *automaticity*, is self inflicted, at a rate of depolarisation corresponding to the discharge rate of the SA node (the natural pacemaker of the heart).

There are other unique and less well understood properties of the conduction system of the heart, e.g. the sequence of myocardial polarisation is opposite to that of depolarisation. Repolarisation commences from the epicardial to the endocardial surface of the heart whilst depolarisation commences from the endo to epicardial surface. The heart being a hollow asymmetrical organ, irregular in shape with unique conduction pathways, it is not difficult to expect the recordings of the distribution of electrical energy through it also to be unique.

THE NORMAL ECG PATTERN

The normal cyclic electrocardiographic pattern of each heart beat consists of five waves known as P, Q, R, S, and T respectively; each of these waves corresponding to different electrical propagations within the heart.

The site of origin is the *sino-atrial node* situated within the right atrium at the junction of the superior vena cava. This structure is one of numerous specialised "automatic" cells that are capable of spontaneous depolarisation depending upon their own intrinsic rate of discharge. Because the sino-atrial node depolarises at a rate higher than any of the other automatic cells it normally has control of the heart rate and is sometimes referred to as the "pacemaker" of the heart.

Once the SA node has depolarised (which produces no discernible signal on the ECG tracing), the surrounding myocardial cells immediately respond until the whole of the right and left atria are depolarised, producing the *"P" wave*. This process is often wrongly described as being a ripple effect similar to that seen when an object is thrown into a still pond, however, there are specialised conduction pathways within the right atrium. These are known as the anterior, posterior and middle internodal tracts. Arising from the anterior internodal tract is *Bachmann's bundle* which is believed to conduct the impulse from the right to the left atrium.

FIGURE 2

The complexes and time intervals of the normal electrocardiogram

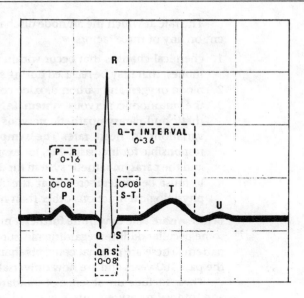

FIGURE 3

Anatomy of the conductive network of the heart

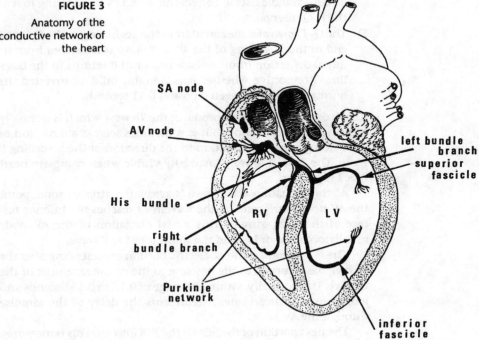

The rate at which the SA node discharges its impulse is dependent on any of three factors:

1. chemical changes that occur within the bloodstream. e.g. hormones, that may be released during stress or emotion, or drugs;
2. blood oxygen and carbon dioxide concentration;
3. the autonomic nervous system (ANS) involving the sympathetic and parasympathetic nervous systems; both controlling variations in heart rate. The sympathetic system is mainly responsible for increases due, for example, to exercise or fright, and the parasympathetic system for decreases e.g. when resting. It must be remembered that the ANS controls many other physiological functions other than heart rate.

Before we are able to venture further it must be noted that there are some peculiar oddities regarding measurement analysis of the ECG pattern. These are original concepts that have not changed during the past 100 years and are now universally accepted.

These include the absence of standards of some of the segment and interval measurements. e.g:

❏ The *P–R interval* is measured from the beginning of the P to the beginning of the Q. There is, however, a tendency by some electro-cardiologists to correct this anomaly by referring to it as the P–Q interval.

❏ The *Q–T interval* is measured from the beginning of the Q to the end of the T! Timing of the atrial P wave is measured from its initial deflection from the base line until it returns to the baseline, irrespective whether it is upright, bifid or inverted. Its normal range is between 0.06 and 0.11 seconds.

Repolarisation of the atria produces the *Ta wave* which is normally hidden from view although it is sometimes seen as a deviation of the P–R segment in opposition to the direction of the preceding P wave. The atrial T wave is markedly visible when complete heart block is present.

As the excitation wave spreads across the atria, at some point the AV node is triggered as the wavefront reaches the inferior surface of the right atrium. This initial excitation of the AV node usually occurs at or beyond the summit of the P wave.

The *P–R segment* is the isoelectric portion commencing after the P wave has returned to the baseline to the commencement of the Q wave. It is normally within the range of 0.12 to 0.15 seconds and lengthens with heart rate. It represents the delay of the impulse through the AV node.

The next portion of the ECG is the *P–R interval*. This is measured from the time the P wave departs from the zero baseline until the onset of the Q wave, or until the first deflection of the QRS departs from the baseline. Although traditionally known as the P–R interval, it is the P–Q interval that is measured and indicates the time during which excitation is delayed as it passes through the AV node, i.e. from the initial onset of atrial excitation until the ventricular septum is excited as the impulse passes through the bundle of His. The normal range of the PR interval is 0.12 to 0.21 s and varies with heart rate and age.

The *QRS complex* is generated as the excitation process rapidly passes through the main *bundle of His*, into the right and left branches and deep into the *Purkinje fibres*. It represents the invasion and subsequent depolarisation of (a) the ventricular septum from left to right, (b) the apex of the heart and (c) the mass of the right and left ventricular walls, commencing at endocardial level and proceeding through the muscle to the epicardial surface.

REMEMBER

> *The most dominant electrical forces are created by the left ventricle* which has a wall thickness some three times that of the right, causing the resultant electrical forces to be directed downwards and towards the left.

The last portions of the ventricular myocardium to be depolarised are usually the right ventricular outflow tract and the superior wall of the left ventricle, giving rise to the *S wave*. The duration of the QRS complex is measured from the initial deflection of the Q wave as it deviates from the baseline until the return of the S wave to the baseline. The normal width is less than 0.10 seconds and is often much narrower in young children (± 0.06). It is important to remember that the first upward deflection of the QRS complex is always known as the R wave.

After depolarisation is complete there is a period of electrical inactivity causing the ECG recording signal to remain on the baseline. This period, known as the *ST segment*, is the part of the electrocardiogram that is most rate dependent and its deviation from the baseline is an important indicator of ischaemic disease. It is measured from the point of return of the S wave to the baseline to the onset of the T wave.

The *T wave* represents the repolarisation of the ventricles and is not accompanied by any physical movement. It is the state when the myocardial cells are depleted of sodium ions and regain their negative charge. Because repolarisation occurs from the epicardium to the endocardium (possibly related to intramural pressure) its polarity is usually positive *(except in lead aVR)* and in the same direction as the QRS complex. Normal inversion of the T wave may be present in lead V1 and is not uncommonly seen in leads V2 and V3 as a normal variant in patients under the age of 30 years.

The *QT-interval* is measured from the beginning of the Q wave to the end of the T wave, i.e. the point where it returns to the baseline. It is significantly affected by heart rate to which it is inversely and exponentially proportional. This means the higher the rate the shorter the Q–T interval and the lower the rate the longer the interval. The relationship is *not* a linear one, i.e. doubling of the rate does not halve the Q–T interval, but is exponentially related.

The normal range of Q–T interval approximates 0.30 to 0.40 seconds for a heart rate of 60–100 bpm and rarely exceeds 0.44 seconds unless the heart rate is excessively slow.

$$\text{Normal QT} = 0.39\sqrt{RR} \pm 10\,\%$$

Because of the non-linear relationship between the QT interval and heart rate and in order to obtain the maximum limits of normal, it is important to arithmetically correct the interval in respect to rate. Possibly the most commonly used formula is that of Bazett:

$$\text{Corrected QT (QTc)} = \frac{QT}{\sqrt{RR}}$$

In the higher limits of heart rate, females usually have slightly longer intervals than males.

Following the T wave a small deflection, usually of the same polarity as the T wave, is sometimes seen, known as the *U wave*. Its origin is uncertain, although believed to be due to repolarisation of a papillary muscle. In certain pathological conditions (e.g. hypokalaemia and cardiac enlargement) it may be pronounced and is often seen in the bradycardic heart.

The 12-lead electrocardiogram

The method of recording the electrocardiogram (ECG) is today universally accepted, although its origins date to the latter part of the last century.

It was Einthoven who in 1903 designated three electrocardiographic "leads", 1, 2 and 3:

❑ Lead 1 was the electrocardiogram he obtained when recording the potential difference between the right (negative) and left (positive) arms.

❑ Lead 2 between the right arm (negative) and the left leg (positive).

❑ Lead 3 between the left arm (negative) and the left leg (positive).

❑ These three leads are commonly known as: *standard limb leads* or bipolar limb leads, each having two poles. Einthoven supposed that the algebraic sum of the amplitude of the QRS complexes in these three leads equalled zero. His theory of the hearts excitation being contained within an equilateral triangle, the corners of which were the shoulders and the pubis, allowed the direction of the electrical forces to be measured.

FIGURE 4

The equalateral triangle of Einthoven depicting the connections of the three bi-polar limb leads 1,2 & 3.

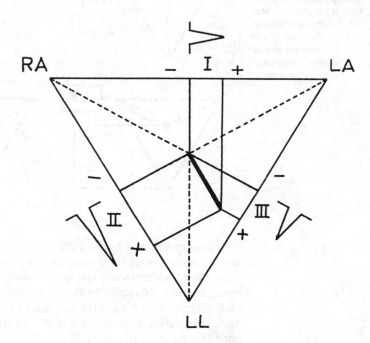

In the year 1942 Goldburger described three leads that increased the value of the standard limb leads, which he named *augmented unipolar limb leads*. They were derived from the three bipolar limb leads with the exception that two of the limbs were electrically connected, and were designated aVR, aVL and aVF, meaning Augmented Vector Right, Left and Foot. The word vector simply relates to something that has magnitude and direction and the letters R, L and F to the right arm, left arm and foot.

Lead aVR is obtained by electrically connecting the left arm and the left leg together, the mid point acting as one pole (negative) and the right arm the other pole (positive).

Lead aVL is obtained in a similar fashion by connecting the right arm and the left leg together (negative) and the left arm the other pole.

In lead aVF the right and left arms are connected (negative pole) and the left leg is the positive pole.

The six limb leads 1,2,3, aVR, aVL and aVF are said to be recorded in the frontal plane, i.e. they are seen as a cross-sectional view at the front of the body.

FIGURE 5

The connections of the
Goldburger
Augmented Unipolar
limb leads aVR, aVL and
aVF and those of Wilson
V1,V2,V3,V4,V5 & V6.
The oblong blocks
represent electrical
resistors.

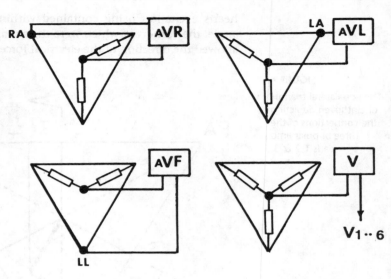

The *unipolar chest leads* of Wilson (1944), commonly known as the *V leads* or Vector leads are created by electrically connecting all three limbs, which by the law of Kirchhoff, will produce a point of zero potential; this point being the indifferent pole of the electrocardiogram, neither negative nor positive, and the other "exploring" pole taken from an electrode located on one of the six positions on the anterior surface of the chest wall. These leads are sometimes referred to as *precordial leads or chest leads.*

The electrocardiogram obtained from these various electrode connections depends entirely on the propagation pattern of the electrical forces that are discharged from the heart to the immediate area of the chest underlying the electrode. Unlike the limb leads, these leads allow cardiac activity to be measured in the horizontal plane, i.e. seen looking down upon a horizontal section of the torso.

As we look at a building from different horizontal directions and obtain different views, so do we obtain different pattern changes of the electrical conduction system of the heart by placing electrodes at different sites on the body. We "see" the spread of excitation from different vantage points.

Figure 6 shows how the resultant electrical forces, represented by the thick arrow, are seen from eight vantage points A to H. The electrograms recorded from sites C, D and E are positive as the forces approach them. Sites G, H and A will produce negative electrograms as the forces are moving away from them, whilst the electrograms recorded from sites B and F are isoelectric as the resultant forces are at right angles to their direction. Sites opposite each other will record equal amplitudes of opposing directions. In a similar way the 12-lead electrocardiogram allows the conduction process to be recorded from twelve vantage points.

FIGURE 6

The excitation patterns of leads as seen from eight different vantage points. The thick arrow represents the electrical axis of the heart.

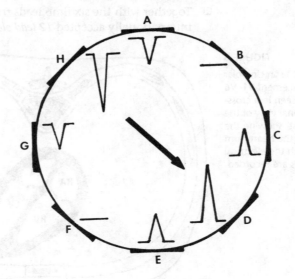

FIGURE 7

The standard chest positions of the six Wilson or Vector (V) Veads (see text)

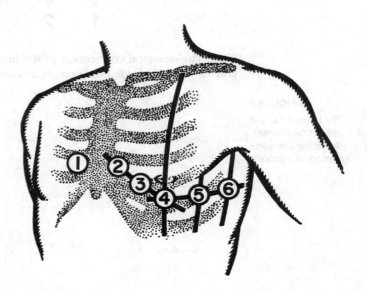

The six areas are V1, V2, V3, V4, V5 and V6, located as follows:

- ❏ V1 = 4th right intercostal space to the right of the sternum
- ❏ V2 = 4th left intercostal space to the left of the sternum.
- ❏ V3 = centrally located between V2 and V4

- ❑ V4 = 5th intercostal space in the mid-clavicular line
- ❑ V5 = lateral to V4 in the anterior axillary line
- ❑ V6 = lateral to V4 and V5 in the mid axillary line.
- ❑ Together with the six limb leads these six V leads complete the internationally accepted *12 lead electrocardiogram.*

FIGURE 8

The Wilson Unipolar lead placement V1–V6 as seen in a cross-sectional view of the chest, showing the areas of the heart from which the electrical forces are recorded.

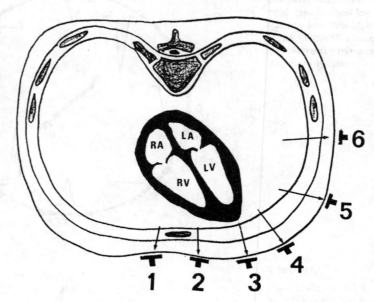

Note: The electrical connection of the limbs when aVR, aVL, aVF and V1–V6 are recorded is automatically done in the ECG machine.

FIGURE 9

The normal 12-lead electrocardiogram. Note the complete inversion of lead aVR.

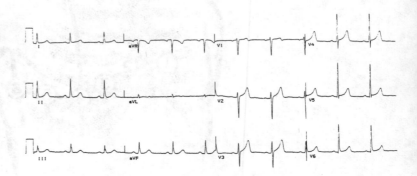

Other leads that are *uncommonly* used include:

- ❑ *V7* = lateral to V4, V5 and V6 in the posterior axillary line.
- ❑ *Oe* = a lead located at the distal portion of an electrode that is introduced into the oesophagus and used for the recording of the electrogram of the adjacent atria. Connection of the proxi-

mal end of the conductive electrode is usually to the central end of one of the "V" leads.

❑ V4R = 4th right intercostal space, mild clavicular line.

❑ *Intracavity* = A unipolar endocardial electrode whose distal end is positioned within a heart chamber and is connected in a similar fashion as the Oe lead i.e. the proximal end to the central terminal of one of the "V" leads.

FIGURE 10

The intra-cavity electrograms of the right atrium (lower left) and the right ventricle (lower right). Obtained by placing an electrically conductive catheter within the respective chambers and using the central terminal of Wilson as one pole and one of the exploring V leads as the other. Shown with the surface electrocardiogram (upper).

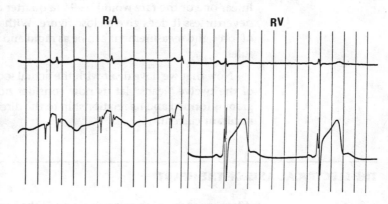

Measurement of heart rate

A convenient method of measuring heart rate from the electrocardiogram tracing is with the use of an ECG ruler. An arrowed cursor is aligned to coincide with the R wave of one ECG complex and a measurement taken after the following second (or third) R wave. Should an ECG ruler not be available it is simple to calculate heart rate by noticing the interval between two adjacent complexes. It must be assumed that the paper speed of the ECG recording mechanism is accurately set at 25 mm/s.

First, find an R wave that is superimposed on a 0.2 second heavy time line of the ECG paper. (The fine lines are 0.04 seconds apart). Then count each of the heavy time lines that follow and mentally designate them as 300, 150, 100, 75, 60, 50, 43 and 37. Should the patient's next R wave coincide with the following heavy time line then the heart rate would be 300. If, however, it coincides with the fourth heavy time line the rate would be 75, and so on.

By this method an accurate heart rate can only be measured if the second R wave is coincident with a 0.2 second line. Should it fall between two lines, which is more than likely, a fair approximation can be made by noticing to which of the lines it is closest. For example, let us assume the second R wave falls a quarter way past 3rd heavy line i.e. between the 100 and 75 lines, the heart rate

FIGURE 11

A simple method of determining heart rate

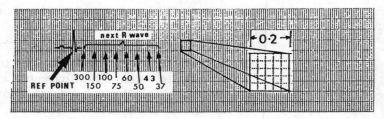

would be 92. It must be remembered that the relationship is not a linear one or the rate would be 94 (a quarter of the difference) but nevertheless it does give a close figure. With practice this method of `on sight' measurement can be as rapid and accurate as your ECG ruler.

Now that we have dealt with the actual location and derivation of the twelve "leads" let us now consider how the electrocardiogram is formed and its relationship to the direction or vector of the resultant current.

THE ELECTRICAL AXIS OF THE HEART

When we speak of the electrical axis of the heart we usually refer to the direction of the electrical forces that are created during the process of depolarisation of the ventricles.

The resultant axis is the summation of all the numerous axes that are generated within the myocardium of the ventricles as they depolarise, and is known as the *mean QRS vector*. Alternatively we may, but actually seldom refer to the axes of the P wave (atrial depolarisation), or more frequently, the T wave (ventricular repolarisation).

Because (a) the physical location of the heart — on the left side pointing downwards and slightly to the left; (b) the origin of the vector is the AV node; and (c) the left ventricle is dominant, one might expect that the electrical axis (or vector) be directed downward and to the left.

Study of the vector forces of the ECG leads allows the axis to be approximately determined.

Let us consider for example the ECG lead 1.

This bipolar limb lead has electrode connections to the patient's right (negative) and left arm (positive) respectively and will give a measurement of the electrical forces generated by the heart that are projected towards it. As the mean QRS vector is acting towards the

FIGURE 12

The mean QRS vector in relation to the three standard limb lead. The central point within the triangle represents the origin of ventricular excitation, i.e. the AV node.

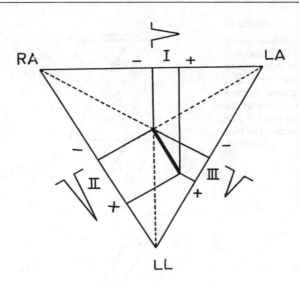

positive pole of the lead at an angle of some 45 % downwards, it will be recorded as an upward deflection, the amplitude of which is dependent upon the angle at which the particular lead sees the vector forces.

When the resultant current vector is parallel and in the same direction as the lead axis, then the deflection of the recorder will be in an upward direction of large amplitude, e.g. the normal lead 2. Conversely, when the vector is parallel but directed in opposition to the lead axis then the recorder deflection will be in a downward direction, e.g. lead aVR. Should, however, the current vector be perpendicular to the lead axis, and directed either towards or away from it, then there will be NO deflection of the recording mechanism. There will also be no deflection should there be absence of current flow. It follows therefore that a current flow that presents itself obliquely to the lead axis will deflect either upwards or downwards depending upon the angle and direction of obliqueness.

Recording the 12 leads of the diagnostic electrocardiogram allows the physician to view the resultant excitation potentials from different vantage points, in a similar way that he would listen to different heart sounds by placing his stethoscope on the various areas on the chest wall, or would position an echocardiograph transducer to beam through acceptable windows of the chest wall.

The measurement of axis The axis or direction is measured in degrees in the frontal plane, completing a circle from 0 to +180 degrees clockwise and 0 to –180 degrees anticlockwise, where zero degree is positioned laterally to the right of the circle, i.e. the patient's left when superimposed on

FIGURE 13

Illustration showing how the QRS pattern is derived in relation to the mean vector and lead direction. The thick arrow represents the vector and the thin arrows the lead direction.

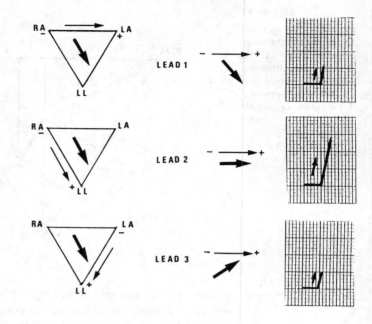

FIGURE 14

The ECG patterns of the augmented limb leads assuming the QRS vector to be 45 degrees. In aVR the mean vector is directed away from the right shoulder, hence the large inverted pattern. In aVL the vector is almost at right angles to the left shoulder, producing a small upright recording. In aVF the vector is towards the positive pole of the left leg, producing a medial upright recording.

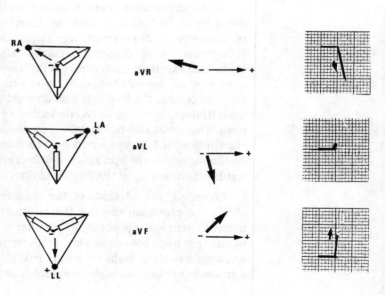

the Einthoven triangle. This is another "oddity" of electro-cardiography in that the circle is not conventionally designated from 0 to 360 degrees The student must be careful not to confuse polarity of the lead direction with the negativity and positivity of the hexaxial system.

FIGURE 15

The limits of the normal mean QRS vector lie between –30 and +105 degrees.

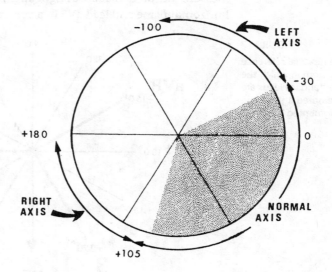

FIGURE 16

In order to determine the algebraic sum of the QRS lead , each of the deflections must be added to or subtracted from each other. In this instance it is
4 – 1 – 3.5 = –0.5

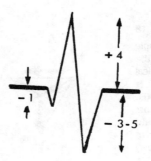

The *normal frontal axis* of the heart extends between –30 and +105 degrees. There is much indecision and dispute regarding the absolute values of normality, but little doubt that an axis greater than +105 degrees would be classified as *right axis deviation (RAD)* and greater than –30 degrees would be *left axis deviation (LAD)*.

In order to measure the electrical axis of the heart it is necessary to determine the algebraic sum of the QRS complexes of each of the leads used. This involves adding all the positive components and subtracting all the negative components of each particular lead. Although it is possible to roughly determine the axis by the measurement of any two of the limb leads, a much more accurate method is to look at all the limb leads.

The *hexaxial reference system* involves the inspection of all six frontal plane leads and particularly leads 1 and aVF. These two leads measure the forces that are at right angles to each other, lead 1 in a horizontal plane and lead aVF in a vertical plane.

FIGURE 17

The hexaxial reference system in which the standard leads are measured against the augmented lead aVF.

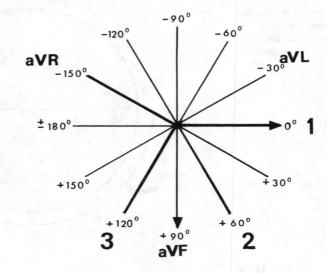

FIGURE 18

(A) Einthovens triangle illustrating the horizontal and vertical positions of leads 1 & aVF .
(B) The equivalent cross vector of leads 1 and aVF showing the axis of 120 degrees (arrow) derived from the respective amplitudes of leads 1 and aVF (C).

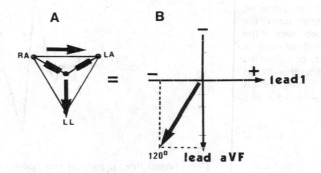

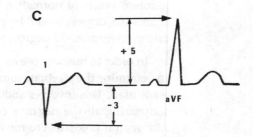

As a rough guide, axes can be measured by determining the lead that has the highest QRS amplitude (either positive or negative). If positive, then that lead will be in the direction determined from the hexaxial reference shown in figure 17.

The following criteria will allow the axis to be quickly determined:

1. If the QRS complexes are upward (positive) in leads 1, 2, 3 and AVf, then the axis *must* be within normal limits.

2. If the QRS complex in lead 1 is downward (negative), and upward (positive) in lead AVf, the axis MUST be greater than +90 and less than +180 (right axis deviation when greater than +105 degrees).

3. If the QRS complex in lead 1 is downward (negative) and also downward (negative) in lead AVf then the axis *must* be greater than +180 degrees i.e. extreme right axis deviation.

4. If the QRS complexes in lead 3 and AVf are downward (negative) then the axis must be greater than 0 degrees, i.e. moderate left axis deviation.

5. If the QRS complex in lead 3 is downward (negative) and upward (positive) in lead AVf then the axis *must* be less than 30 degrees, i.e. mild left axis deviation.

6. If the QRS complexes in leads 3, AVf and 2 are downward (negative) the axis *must* be greater than –30 degrees, i.e. moderate to severe left axis deviation. An axis deviation greater than –90 degrees is very uncommon.

7. Should the QRS complex in any of the limb leads be biphasic and of equal deflection, i.e. the upward component is exactly the same amplitude as its downward component, then the axis must be perpendicular to that lead direction. For example, should the algebraic sum of the deflections in lead 2 equal or near equal zero, the axis must be either –30 or +150 degrees.

Axis deviation Right axis deviation is commonly seen in any condition of dominance of the right ventricle, chronic lung disease, congenital heart disease, cor pulmonale, pulmonary embolism, pulmonary hypertension, RVH due to any cause, anterolateral myocardial infarction, left posterior hemiblock, WPW etc.

Left axis deviation is seen in ischaemic heart disease, aortic stenosis, congenital heart disease, systemic hypertension, LVH due to any cause, inferior wall infarction, left anterior hemiblock, pacemaking, WPW etc.

Note: It should be realised, however, that measurement of the axis of the heart by any means that accepts the hypothesis of Einthoven cannot be considered to have great accuracy. After practice the student will soon be able to give a good approximation of the axis of the ventricles by relating the degree of negativity or positivity of the leads in question.

P wave axis The P wave axis determines the direction of atrial depolarisation. When the origin of excitation is the SA node then the axis is normally shown by upright P waves in all limb leads except aVR, the P wave axis directed downward and to the left (15–75 degrees). However, when the site of origin is other than the SA node then the term *"non-sinus rhythm"* is used and frequently causes inversion or absence of the P waves. It seems logical that an ectopic rhythm originating in the lower part of the atrium would produce an inverted P wave due to retrograde conduction and as such the axis might be reversed.

The T wave axis is normally of the same direction as the QRS complex and its axis directed downward and to the left.

The mean horizontal axis of the heart may be determined in a similar way as the mean frontal axis using a hexaxial system of the six Wilson V leads.

THE ABNORMAL ELECTROCARDIOGRAM

Before the abnormalities of the electrocardiogram are discussed it is important to be familiar with a method of study of each of the waveforms of the ECG. By answering questions the student is able to draw conclusions and determine the normalities and abnormalities of the conduction system. As the excitation normally proceeds from the sino-atrial node it seems logical to commence at that point:

1. What is the RATE? Is there:
   - bradycardia (< 60) or
   - tachycardia (> 100)?
2. The P waves — are they:
   - normal in contour?
   - abnormally tall?
   - wide or bifid?
   - absent or inverted?
   - followed by and related to a QRS complex? i.e.1:1 rhythm
   - identical in any given lead?
   - regular?
3. The P–R interval — is it:
   - shortened? (< 0.12 s)
   - lengthened? (> 0.21 s)
   - non-existent?
4. The QRS complexes — are they:
   - large or small in amplitude?

- widened? (> 0.11 s)
- bifid?
- abnormally inverted?
- regular?

are there:

- large Q waves — S waves?

what is the:

- mean frontal axis?
- rate?

5. The S–T segment — is there:
- depression?
- elevation?

6. The T waves — are they:
- tall and peaky?
- flat?
- inverted?
- directed away from the QRS?
- small?

7. The Q–T interval — is it:
- shortened?
- lengthened?

Then, determine the rhythm.

Normal variants   Normal variants of the electrocardiographic pattern may be seen that are related to:

❑ *Age.* The P wave of the newborn child is often tall and peaky and short in duration. The P–R interval is short in duration although not normally less than 0.07 seconds. The QRS complex is narrow and there is almost always right axis deviation. The T waves are variable and tachycardia is characteristic in the infant electrocardiogram.

❑ As childhood advances the P–R interval lengthens and the axis becomes normal; throughout early life there is a progressive change of pattern from one of RV dominance to LV dominance with an intermediate balanced situation. The QRS slightly lengthens. As age advances, the P–R interval increases, the QRS varies due to varying thickness of the heart muscle and in old age the T wave flattens and the axis becomes directed posteriorly.

❑ *Build.* Tall thin people usually have thin or pendulous hearts, whilst short fat people have fat or squat hearts, each type producing alteration of the electrical axis. The pendulous heart produces a pattern of right axis deviation (RAD) and the squat heart a left axis deviation (LAD). Obese people and pregnant women are likely to have LAD because of the upward lift of the diaphragm and rotation of the heart to the left. A deep Q may be seen in lead 3.

❑ *Athletes* often have large hearts with tall QRS and T waves ("athletic heart") associated with marked sinus or junctional bradycardia at rest, long P–R intervals outside the normal range, and often accompanied with left ventricular hypertrophy and other ECG abnormalities.

❑ *Posture* may considerably alter the ECG pattern whether it be due to anatomical displacement or disease.

❑ *Breathing* causes the heart rate to slow during expiration and quicken during inspiration. It also slightly alters the electrical axis of the heart as the diaphragm is raised and lowered.

Now let us relate some of the deformities of the ECG complexes and intervals with pathological conditions. At this point it is important to remember that the electrocardiogram is a recording of the propagation of the *resultant electrical forces* through the heart muscle. It does *not* give information per se of pathological or mechanical dysfunction, but abnormal features are often correlated to them.

ENLARGEMENT OR HYPERTROPHY OF THE CHAMBERS

The right atria

Tall, peaky P waves (> 2.5 mm) in leads 2, 3 and AVf, (sometimes known as "P pulmonale"), with tall or biphasic P waves in the right sided V leads are characteristic of right atrial enlargement. This abnormality is often associated with chronic lung disease, tricuspid valve or congenital heart disease.

The left atria

The P wave is widened, (> 0.12 s) and biphasic in leads 1, 2 and V1, with a prominent negative portion in lead V1. It may be negative in leads 3 and Avf.

The feature of bilateral atrial enlargement is a combination of both patterns.

The right ventricle

Perhaps the most important features of right ventricular hypertrophy (RVH) are associated with the QRS complexes. The normal ECG pattern and axis is governed to a large extent by the mass of left ventricular muscle. Should, however, the right ventricle become dominant it can be expected that the direction and axis of the QRS complexes will be affected. In the right precordial leads V1 and V2 there is marked increase in the amplitude of the R waves with T wave inversion. The S–T segment in these leads are depressed with an upward convexity. Conspicuous S waves are present in leads V4, V5 and V6, signifying the abnormally large depolarisation signals that are directed away from that part of the chest. The QRS width is within normal limits, but may be slightly increased and there is usually dominant right axis deviation (> 105 degrees). Occasionally a P pulmonale may be present.

The left ventricle

Hypertrophy of the left ventricle always exaggerates the electrical dominance of the ECG pattern. There is an increased QRS amplitude in the limb leads. The QRS complexes are often widened to the upper limits of normal (or beyond) due to the larger mass of muscle through which the excitation process must traverse.

The R waves in leads V5 and V6 are usually large and the S waves in V1 and V2 are deep.

The S–T segment may be depressed with an upward convexity and the T waves are always inverted in leads V5 and V6. The axis is shifted to the left (LAD) (> –30 degrees) and there is often left atrial enlargement.

Right and left ventricles (bi-ventricular)

This ECG diagnosis is often difficult as hypertrophy of one chamber is seen to be cancelled out by the hypertrophy of the other which may produce a "pseudo normal" ECG.

The amplitude of the QRS complexes satisfy both RVH and LVH, often showing equiphasic complexes in the precordial leads V3 and V4. There may be ECG dominance of one of the ventricular chambers with discordance of the axis and incomplete bundle branch block.

FIGURE 19
Characteristic hypertrophy patterns. Note the marked amplitude of the R waves in V1,V2 and V3 in the RVH pattern. In LVH there are large amplitude R waves in the limb leads and tall R waves with T wave inversion in leads V5 and V6 (see text).

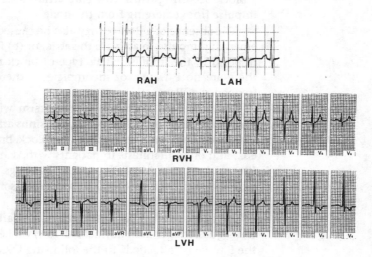

23

Conduction dysfunction Dysfunction of the process of conduction is commonly seen in the normal heart and are usually short lived benign anomalies e.g. bradycardia, VPBs etc, that produce minor palpitations. On the other hand there are many other abnormalities that cause rhythm disturbance which may minimally affect the well-being of the patient or may be life-threatening, with several symptomatic variations in between.

HEART BLOCKS

Heart block is the condition when any organic lesion or functional disturbance impedes, either partially (incompletely) or completely, the normal conduction process. It may involve any part or parts of the excitation process.

Intra-atrial block (occurring within the atria) is characterised by widened P waves (> 0.12 s) with or without notching. The ECG diagnosis may sometimes be confused with atrial enlargement.

FIGURE 20

Sino-atrial block. Note the absence of P waves due to the failure of the SA node to discharge an impulse.

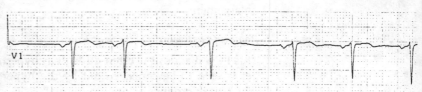

In *S–A block* there is an absence of P waves which generally signifies either the inability of the node to produce an impulse, or a block occurring within the sino-atrial node which prevents the impulse from emerging from the node.

The absence of a P wave may also be caused by (a) failure of the emerging impulse to activate the atria, or (b) failure of the atria to respond to the impulse.[1] This type of block may be complete — there are no P waves, or incomplete — there is an intermittent frequency of P waves.

The *sick sinus syndrome*, a vague term which includes many varieties of sinus node depression, e.g. sinus arrest, prolonged sinus pauses, extreme sinus bradycardia, SA block, brady-tachy syndrome etc., and often manifests in patients with ischaemic heart disease. It may also be temporarily induced by drugs. Many electrophysiologists believe the syndrome to be a precursor to a more advanced grade of heart block.

First-degree A–V block (HB1) may be clearly seen on the ECG tracing as a longer than normal P–R interval i.e. > 0.21secs. Because the P wave is "attached" to the following QRS complex, the block is incomplete due to an abnormal delay of conduction at the AV node, although the block may occur within the internodal pathways, His bundle, or even within one of the branches of the His if the other branch is blocked. If there were no QRS complexes following, other than those that occasionally and randomly occur, there wõuld be a complete blockage of conduction.

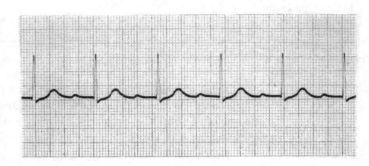

Second-degree A–V block (HB2) is a form of incomplete block of two distinct types:

Mobitz type 1 A–V block is characterised by a progressive lengthening of the P–R interval and is due to a block within the A–V junction. There is a progressive decrease in the conduction velocity until the impulse fails to conduct to the ventricles. Known as the *Wenckebach phenomenon*, the P–R interval usually begins within normal limits and gradually lengthens with each successive beat until a ventricular beat is dropped, after which the normal P–R interval is resumed and the sequence repeated. Figure 22 shows two dropped beats although typically only one is usually dropped.

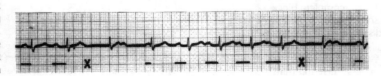

Mobitz type 2 A–V block is characterised by the presence of at least two consecutive normally conducted beats that are followed by a dropped beat and is due to a block usually situated below the bundle of His. The "dropped" beats are caused by intermittent block of the other bundle branch i.e. bilateral bundle branch block and may occur occasionally or in an atrial/ventricular ratio of 2:1, 3:1, 4:1. Frequently the QRS complexes resemble a bundle branch block pattern, which intermittently progresses to a bilateral branch block, so causing the dropped beats. This type of block is usually a forerunner to complete heart block.

FIGURE 23

Mobitz type 2 high grade second degree heart block in which each third beat is blocked at or distal to the AV node.

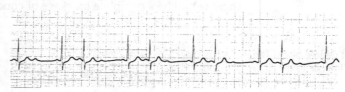

Third-degree (HB3) or *complete heart block* (CHB) is characterised by a complete dissociation of the P waves and the QRS complexes. None of the impulses originating from the atria are responsible for ventricular activation.

The cause is complete block of conduction either at the AV junction (type 1), the bundle of His, both bundle branches or at fascicular level (type 2). This is the most serious form of block and may provoke prolonged ventricular standstill and subsequent death. Commonly the patient is seen to have a characteristic fit, known as a *Stokes–Adams attack* (or Adams–Stokes) immediately after the commencement of the heart block. However, a secondary pacemaker such as the A–V node or some ventricular foci will often respond, producing either an *A–V junctional escape rhythm* or a ventricular escape rhythm and discharge at a low rate preventing the immediate risk. This slow ventricular rate or *idioventricular rhythm,* is usually around 40 bpm but may be as low as 10 or as high as 60 in the infant. If permanent in nature the effective treatment may call for the implantation of a cardiac pacemaker.

FIGURE 24

Third degree heart complete block showing the complete dissociation of the atria and ventricles. The P waves preceding the first and third complexes are purely coincidental.

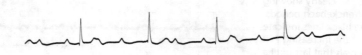

Bundle branch blocks Functional or organic disturbance of the bundle of His and its branches, including the musculature of the ventricles produces a partial or complete cessation of the excitation stimulus beyond the affected area. The QRS complexes show characteristic notching and widening. Electrical blockage of one of the two bifurcations of the main bundle of His, known respectively as the right and left branches, creates an abnormal conduction process to the chamber that is blocked. The most common cause of bundle branch block is idiopathic degenerative disease; of the two branches it is the right branch that is most commonly affected.

Should there be *right bundle branch block* (RBBB), conduction can only proceed through the left bundle branch, which would depolarise the left ventricle in a normal manner and belatedly depolarise the right ventricle via impulses that spread through the septum. The ECG pattern characteristically shows notching and widening of the QRS complexes especially seen in the right sided chest leads. This notching, or bifurcation, and widening of the QRS complexes may be readily understood if it is realised that the right ventricle is depolarised after the left, each producing their R waves on the ECG as they depolarise, (the R–S–R pattern). The QRS duration is normally > 0.11 seconds. Should the notching of the QRS complexes be associated with normal widening, i.e. < 0.90 seconds, it must be presumed that the block is not complete and generally termed an *RV conduction defect* or *incomplete RBBB*.[2]

Right axis deviation is common, wide S waves are seen in the precordial leads and ventricular activation time is increased beyond 0.03 seconds.

FIGURE 25

Right bundle branch block. (Limb leads upper, chest leads lower) Note the notching seen in the right-sided chest leads V1 to V3.

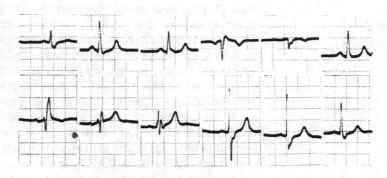

Should *left bundle branch block* (LBBB) develop, the excitation impulse will travel through the right bundle, where it will depolarise the right ventricle in the normal manner and belatedly depolarise the left ventricle across the ventricular septum. In a similar way that the right ventricle is affected in RBBB, notching may be seen in the left sided chest leads. Widening (> 0.12 s) of the QRS complexes is seen in ALL leads and left axis deviation is common. Ventricular activation time is prolonged by 0.05 seconds.

Remember: In normal conduction the septum is excited from left to right. When blockage of the right bundle occurs (RBBB) the septum will still be excited from left to right, and produce a normal initial Q wave of the QRS complex, BUT, when the left branch is blocked (LBBB), there is no longer normal activation of the septum, and no Q waves would be seen in the left chest ECG leads. Because the left ventricle has a far greater mass of muscle than its right counterpart, the mean frontal axis is often unaltered and ST segment changes and T wave inversions are commonly seen with LBBB.

FIGURE 26
Left bundle branch block. Note the widening in all leads.

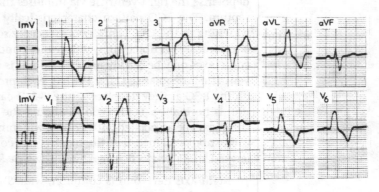

Fascicular blocks

Proceeding from the AV node, the right branch of the His bundle is relatively large in diameter when compared to the left and does not branch until it reaches the right ventricular apex. The left branch of the bundle of His has two conduction fascicles that arise to form the *left anterior fascicle* and the *left posterior fascicle* respectively. (The right bundle branch is regarded as the 3rd fascicle)

Pure block of either or both of these bifurcations does not normally produce more than minimal changes in QRS width, morphology, S–T segment or T wave configuration. The only clue is a massive shift of the QRS axis which is especially large (> –30 degrees) in blockage of the left anterior fascicle, commonly known as a *left anterior hemiblock* (LAHB). In blockage of the left posterior fascicle, known as *left posterior hemiblock* (LPHM), the axis is shifted towards the right (> +120 degrees) simulating RVH. However, block of either of these fascicles is often associated with RBBB which will, in any case, produce abnormally wide QRS complexes. It must be remembered that either form of hemiblock can simulate other pathological conditions such as infarction and hypertrophy. Of the two types, LAH is by far the most common and the most frequent cause of either type is ischaemic heart disease.

When two fascicles are blocked it is generally referred to as *bifascicular block* and when three become blocked it is known as *trifasci-*

cular block. Although this term generally refers to blockage of the right bundle plus the two left fascicles, i.e. complete heart block, it may also include any condition where three blockages occur distal to the A–V node. Lengthening of the P–R interval is often seen in trifascicular block due to prolongation of the normal excitation process.

FIGURE 27
The fascicles of the left bundle branch.

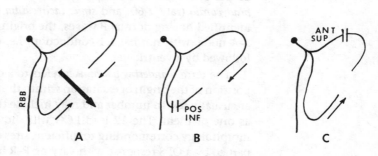

ABNORMAL RHYTHMS

In the broadest sense the word "arrhythmia" relates to any rhythm that is abnormal or absent. There are a few exceptions. Some that are not strictly deviations from normal, e.g., respiratory arrhythmia, and some that are never termed arrhythmias e.g. cardiac standstill.

For all practical purposes abnormalities of cardiac rhythm may be classified into either:

❑ *Supraventricular*: those originating above the bifurcation of the His bundle. or
❑ *Ventricular:* those originating distal to the bifurcation of the His bundle.

In order to distinguish between the two it is important that all leads of the ECG be very carefully examined. It is sometimes difficult to determine, especially when a supraventricular tachycardia with aberration is present. Even expert electrocardiologists are sometimes at a loss to make an ECG diagnosis under such circumstances.

Supraventricular rhythms

Irregularity of the heart beat is commonly due to the presence of a supraventricular rhythm which may take the form of either:

❑ Sinus arrhythmia,
❑ Wandering pacemaker,
❑ Non-sinus atrial rhythm,
❑ Paroxysmal atrial tachycardia (PAT),
❑ Atrial flutter (AFl),

- ❑ Atrial fibrillation (AF),
- ❑ Atrial ectopy (APBs),
- ❑ A–V junctional rhythm

Sinus arrhythmia may be defined as any condition in which the sinus node discharges irregularly at a rate that may vary as much as 25 per cent. The QRS complexes have normal morphology. *sinus bradycardia* (rate < 60) and *sinus tachycardia* (rate > 100) are both identified having normal P waves, the origin of impulse being the S–A node, with normal 1:1 conduction, i.e. each atrial excitation followed by a ventricular.

The term *wandering pacemaker* refers to a continuous change of position of the origin of excitation within the atria. The ectopic foci are usually few in number and may include the natural pacemaker as one of them. The 12 lead ECG will show changes in P wave morphology corresponding to different sites of focus, each accompanied by a QRS response with varying P–R intervals.

Non-sinus atrial rhythm is well recognised by inversion of the P waves with a short P–R interval, signifying a retrograde atrial conduction that originates low in the right atrial chamber.

FIGURE 28
Non-sinus rhythm showing inversion of P waves in leads 2 and 3. The origin of excitation is low within the atrium at or near the AV node causing retrograde conduction of the atria.

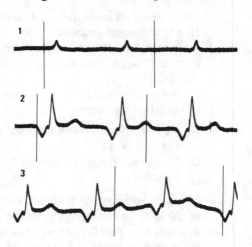

Paroxysmal atrial tachycardia (PAT) is characterised by a rapid ventricular rate somewhere between 160 and 240, each normal QRS complex preceded by a P wave that is usually abnormal in contour and often inverted. When the atrial rate is very high it is often impossible to see the P waves, which become merged within the preceding T wave, often making it extremely difficult to distinguish between PAT and A–V junctional tachycardia. (More often than not, most episodes of PAT are thought to be junctional in origin). The origin of the impulse is usually at an ectopic site within the atrium or may be the result of A–V nodal re-entry.

FIGURE 29

Paroxysmal atrial tachycardia of rate 160 bpm

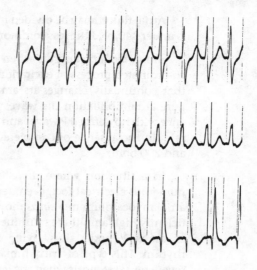

Atrial flutter is a rapid atrial rhythm that is frequently caused by a repetitive discharge of excitatory impulses that originate in the right atrium. The movement of discharge is in the form of a ring, or "circus" that extends between the two venae cavae. This cyclic discharge produces broad P waves, known as *flutter waves,* that merge into each other producing a saw tooth appearance. The resultant QRS complexes do not normally follow each flutter wave and may be conducted alternatively, i.e. 2:1, at a regular rate.

The ventricular rate is high with the 2nd P wave hidden within the QRS and may therefore be confused with sinus, atrial or A–V junctional tachycardia. Atrial flutter may also be present with varying conduction ratios, e.g. 3:1, 4:1, 5:1 etc.

FIGURE 30

Atrial flutter at rate of 250 per minute with a 3:1 and 4:1 variable ventricular response. note the large amplitude variation of right atrial "a" waves.

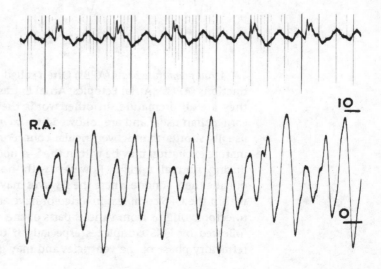

Atrial flutter may be divided into two types: type 1 of a rate that is under 340, and the less common type 2 of rates over 340 (Waldo).

Atrial fibrillation occurs when the atria can no longer sustain a co-ordinated process of excitation resulting in an irregular activity that continually changes its amplitude, shape and direction. In pure atrial fibrillation the waves may be coarse or fine in appearance with no defined P waves and an irregular supraventricular QRS rate (in the absence of complete heart block) varying between 50 and 200 bpm.

In a situation where there is spontaneous depolarisation of numerous electrical foci, each depolarising a small segment of the atrial myocardium in a *circus* movement, resultant impulses of sufficiently high amplitude must inevitable trigger a random response of the A–V node, thus giving rise to the irregular ventricular rhythm. This type of arrhythmia is commonly seen as a result of severe mitral stenosis when the left atrium is enlarged and compromised. A combination of flutter/fib waves may be seen on the ECG baseline as the atria alternate their rhythm between fibrillation and flutter. The flutter waves are often poorly defined in the presence of such a rhythm.

FIGURE 31

Atrial fibrillation with fine fibrillatory waves of low amplitude. Note the irregular excitation of the ventricles

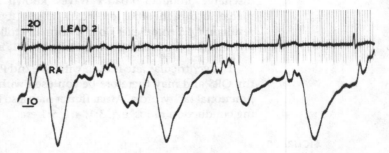

Atrial premature beats (APBs) Often called Atrial Premature Contractions (APCs); Atrial Ectopics; Atrial Extrasystoles, but whatever, they are all premature. In other words they occur unexpectedly earlier than usual and are followed by a *compensatory pause* that is usually shorter than its ventricular counterpart. The origin of premature excitation may be within the S–A node. (Sinus ectopy) producing normal upright P waves with normal morphology or outside the S–A node where the P waves may be absent, i.e. hidden within the QRS complex, inverted or have abnormal contours due to ectopic origins from various parts of the atria. Not all APB's are followed by QRS complexes especially if they occur during the refractory phase of the ventricles and may give rise to a non-conducted bigeminy when every alternate ectopic beat does not conduct to the ventricles.

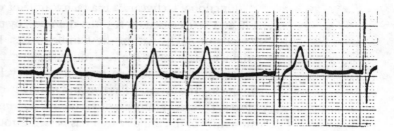

A–V junctional rhythm has its origin in the region of the junction i.e. within or adjacent to the atrio-ventricular node, producing normal antegrade conduction through the ventricles, a normal narrow QRS complex with retrograde conduction through the atria.[3] An inverted P wave may be seen in most leads except aVR. The rate of discharge is usually between 40 and 60 bpm but may be as low as 10 bpm, and can only be sustained as long as the S–A node is ineffective. Because the origin of impulse is no longer from a natural pacemaker it is known as an *escape rhythm*.

The electrical axis of the P wave is usually around –90 degrees, producing a positive P wave in lead aVR and negative in most other leads.

It would be expected that the P(inverted)–R interval be shorter than normal if atrial depolarisation and His bundle conduction occurred simultaneously. This situation is true when the origin of the impulse is high within the A–V node, but should it originate at a lower level, then the inverted P waves may be either absent, i.e. hidden within the QRS complex, or be seen to follow the QRS complex. In the latter instance the ventricles would depolarise before the atria. It must be remembered that conduction through the A–V node whether antegrade or retrograde is normally at a uniform rate. However, should there be a delay in retrograde conduction it would also cause atrial depolarisation to be delayed and produce a P wave after the QRS. Single beats are known as *junctional premature beats* and when a tachycardia is present as *junctional tachycardia*. (The term "A–V nodal" is no longer favoured, due to

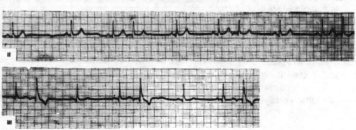

doubt that the A–V node has any pacemaking cells capable of producing stimuli).

Junctional tachycardia is a tachycardia of rate usually between 140 and 180, caused more often than not, by *reentry* within the A–V node or rarely, within the bundle of His. The impulse, whose origin is at or near the A–V node, having taken two pathways known as alpha and beta respectively, recycles within the node producing the inverted P waves and normally conducted QRS complexes. This arrhythmia is often termed a *reentry tachycardia* due to the ability of the impulse that has passed through one of the pathways to return to its site of origin via the other pathway. The condition of reentry is that the second pathway (beta) must possess a unidirectional block that prevents the impulse from travelling in an antegrade manner, but will allow the impulse that travelled down the first (alpha) pathway to return to its site of origin. The atria are therefore retrogradely depolarised causing the tachycardia. In order for the cyclic pattern of conduction to occur there must be two pathways within the A–V node or one pathway plus an *accessory by-pass tract*, as found in the *Wolff–Parkinson–White (WPW)* pre-excitation syndrome.

REMEMBER

□ Supraventricular rhythms, as opposed to ventricular, usually produce *normal narrow QRS complexes.*
□ Tachycardias are generated by three possible mechanisms:
  • repetitive firing of an ectopic impulse within the atrial or ventricular myocardium or within conducting tissue,
  • circus movements as in flutter,
  • reentry of an impulse as described above.
□ Most tachycardias will show S–T segment and/or T wave changes on the ECG due to a lessening of coronary blood flow that is influenced by inadequate diastolic filling.

FIGURE 34

Junctional paroxmysmal tachycardia of rate 138. P–R = 0.1 s. Note inversion of P waves in leads 2 and 3 and spontaneous return to sinus rhythm in leads 1 and 2. (Leads not recorded simultaneously.)

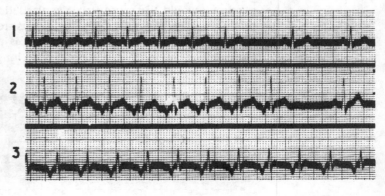

Ventricular rhythms

Ventricular rhythms are those that have not been activated by impulses travelling through the normal ventricular conduction system. The site of electrical activation is from an automatic myocardial cell that may be anywhere within the ventricular myocardium. The result is widened (> 0.10 second) and often bizarre QRS complexes invariably with inversion of the T waves, indicating that excitation took longer than usual to distribute throughout the ventricles, having bypassed the His bundle and Purkinje network. It should be emphasised, however, that not all wide QRS complexes are related to ventricular rhythms, e.g. the bundle branch blocks, WPW or pre-excitation syndrome.

Ventricular aberrations are classified by a host of lexical terms. We read of ventricular premature beats (VPBs); ventricular premature contractions (VPCs); ectopic beats; extrasystoles; parasystoles (not a common term); idioventricular beats; interpolated beats; which to many, all have the same meaning.

All of these are ectopic beats, for they all originate from a source other than the S–A node, but not all ectopic beats are premature, parasystolic or idioventricular. A parasystole is an extrasystole but not all extrasystoles are parasystoles. VPBs and VPCs are the same. Ectopics and extrasystoles may originate in any of the four heart chambers.

The interpreter of the electrocardiogram must be particularly careful when classifying any form of ectopy and must understand the differences. Generally, all premature contractions may be classified as those with *fixed coupling intervals* and those without *fixed coupling intervals*, i.e. with variable coupling which are considered characteristic of rhythms that are automatically initiated and have no relationship to the preceding beat.

The *ventricular premature beat* (VPB), is an early beat that has its origin within the ventricular myocardium and is electrically related to the preceding beat. Its *coupling interval* i.e. the interval between the preceding beat and the VPB, is short and it usually occurs immediately or shortly after the T wave of the preceding beat. It is recognised by a large and wide QRS complex and followed by a *compensatory pause* before the next normal beat is resumed. The time interval between the beat preceding and the beat following the VPB is exactly equal to two normal cardiac cycles (longer than the APB). It is a true extrasystole. P waves may be hidden or seen to appear after the QRS complex indicating retrograde atrial conduction.

The *interpolated beat* is an extrasystole that has occurred very prematurely enabling the ventricle to respond to the next S–A node discharge. The ectopic is therefore seen to squeeze in between two adjacent normal complexes. There are no compensatory pauses.

FIGURE 35

Two examples of
ventricular premature
beats. Note the loss of
pressure within the
ventrical occuring
within each beat.

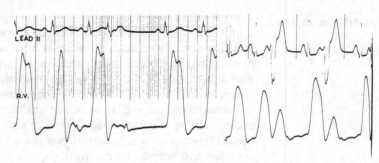

FIGURE 35

Two examples of ventricular premature beats. Note the loss of pressure within the ventrical occuring within each beat.

FIGURE 36

The interpolated beat (see text)

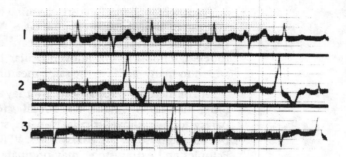

The *ectopic beat* is one that has its focus outside the S–A node and therefore encompasses many ventricular aberrations. It is not, like the VPB, necessarily dependent on the preceding beat.

The *parasystole* is an ectopic beat that is caused by the presence of a secondary "pacemaker", usually in the ventricle, that competes with the SA node at its own independent rate. It is a premature contraction that has no fixed relationship with the preceding conducted beat and is protected by an entry block. It will continue to discharge at its own rate, only appearing as an ectopic beat when the ventricle is refractory, and may be seen as an isolated beat, or, to alternate with a normally conducted beat or beats at regular short intervals depending upon the relationship between the natural and the ectopic rates. Occasionally *fusion beats* may occur when the ectopic impulse occurs late in the cardiac cycle as it periodically coincides with the discharge of the normally conducted beat. Rarely two or more parasystolic rhythms may occur simultaneously, and unlike the ventricular premature beat, the coupling interval of the parasystole is always variable.

The *idioventricular beat* is one that originates from within the ventricular myocardium producing wide QRS complexes that are bizarre with inverted T waves. It is an ectopic beat or rhythm that takes over whenever the sino-atrial and junctional pacemakers fail. Should however it be a repetitive series of beats at a rate of between

20 and 45 beats per minute then it is known as an *idioventricular rhythm*. When the discharge rate is over 100 it is known as an *accelerated idioventricular rhythm*.

Ventricular tachycardia. Often a serious condition that may be considered as a series of idioventricular beats discharging from a single focus at a rate of over 100 bpm. By definition it is a run of at least 3 consecutive and regular beats producing wide bizarre QRS complexes > 14ms. The axis is < 30 degrees

The P waves are unrelated to the QRS and randomly occur during the ectopy. It is not certain whether all ventricular tachycardias emanate from a single source or are created by a reentry within the His-Purkinje or fascicular networks, i.e. *micro-reentry*.

FIGURE 37

Ventricular tachycardia of rate 200. Note the regular repeatable pattern of the paroxysm.

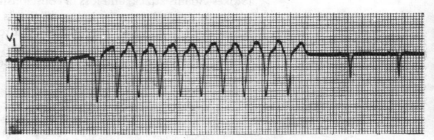

Ventricular flutter is usually seen as a rapid rate that has the appearance of a sinusoidal waveform. Neither QRS nor T waves are defined and the rate is similar to that of ventricular tachycardia.

The *Wolff–Parkinson–White (WPW) syndrome* was first described by these three physicians in 1930 as an electrocardiographic anomaly of a shortened P–R interval with a prolonged QRS duration. It was not until many years later that this ECG malformation was found to be due to an abnormal electrical pathway that connected the atria to the ventricles. As this *accessory pathway* runs perpendicular to the atrio-ventricular ring and conducts at a faster rate than the A–V node, depolarisation of the atria is prematurely conducted to the ventricles, thereby producing the early depolarisation and slurring of the initial QRS complex -the *delta wave* — with a shortened P–R interval. It is very common for the A–V node to also conduct resulting in a fusion of the QRS complex. Tsai and colleagues[4] have described a reliable algorithm based on the polarity of the delta wave and QRS complexes in localising the position of the accessory pathway(s). Be careful, do not confuse with RBBB or LBBB!

Ventricular fibrillation is invariably an irreversible and terminal arrhythmia, except perhaps occasionally in the young healthy heart. It is characteristically shown on the ECG as a series of unco-ordinated irregular chaotic waves that continually vary in both amplitude and frequency. It is caused by multiple re-entry foci within the ventricular myocardium.

FIGURE 38

The electrocardiogram of W–P–W syndrome. Note the delta wave preceding each QRS complex.

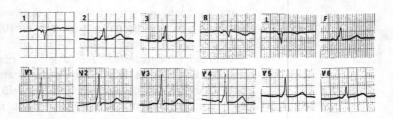

The fibrillating heart is seen to move "like a bag of worms in a plastic bag" producing a loss of blood pressure and cardiac output. The onset is usually followed by sudden fitlike body motions (Stokes–Adams attack) and loss of consciousness, and if allowed to continue, death. It is an "arrhythmia" that is often associated with acute myocardial infarction; coronary artery disease; unstable angina; congenital long Q–T syndrome, and electric shock. Treatment is only effective with the immediate use of a DC defibrillator (q.v.).

FIGURE 39

Ventricular fibrillation

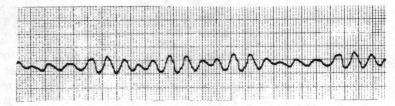

MYOCARDIAL ISCHAEMIA AND INFARCTION

Introduction Most student technologists often find the resultant changes of the electrocardiogram during myocardial anoxia very confusing to understand, despite the extensive reading matter that is available on the subject. It is in itself a complicated subject and the student who wishes to enhance his knowledge may read some of the excellent publications in book form of the more well known electrocardiologists and electrophysiologists. Like all sciences, there are always exceptions to the rule, and there seem to be so many in electrocardiography!

Of all the major ramifications of the coronary circulation, the most prone to occlusion is the left anterior descending branch affecting the anteroseptal and anterior areas of the heart, accounting for near 50 per cent of all infarctions. The second most affected is the right coronary that supplies the diaphragmatic and posterior portions of the heart (30 per cent). The left circumflex supplies the anterolateral, posterolateral and diaphragmatic areas affecting approximately 10 per cent.

It is, of course, not uncommon for both right and left branches of the coronary circulation to be equally affected. Because of the good blood supply to the right atrium and right ventricle via the right and left (anterior descending) coronary arteries, and the low work load and consequent oxygen demand of these two chambers, they are rarely affected.

The electrocardiographic changes that occur when any portion of the myocardium is sufficiently deprived of oxygenated blood affects either the Q waves, S–T segment or the T waves, or any combination of all three.

FIGURE 40

The typical ECG pattern of acute myocardial infarction that is seen in those leads that faced the damaged area. Note the deep, often widened Q wave, the elevated ST segment and the inverted V-shaped T wave.

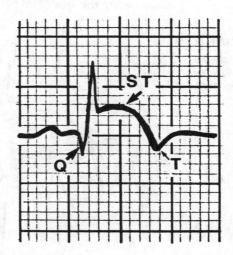

The normal Q wave is the result of septal depolarisation from left to right and is usually small in amplitude (< 25 % of the adjacent R wave) and narrow in width (< 0.04 sec). It is seen on the ECG as a negative deflection in the leads that are directed away from the left ventricle and include 1, aVL, V5 and V6.

However, when the myocardial tissue of the left ventricle is infarcted and necrosis occurs, it cannot generate electrical currents. *It is because of this absence of electrical activity* of the infarcted portion of the left ventricle that causes the depolarisation forces in the right side to be dominant, so producing the large Q waves (> 25 % of R). In assessing infarction from the electrocardiogram the student is advised to carefully determine the presence of recent dominant Q waves, of S–T segment elevations and inversions of T waves. He or she should then make note of the leads that are most affected, remembering that those leads will image the area of infarction.

For example, let us imagine an infarct of the *inferior wall* of the heart (commonly known as *diaphragmatic*, due to a large portion resting on the diaphragm). The leads that positively face the area of infarction are 2, 3 and aVF and therefore would show abnormalities. On the other hand an *anterior wall* infarct would best be seen in leads 1, aVL and the right sided chest leads. *lateral wall* infarction would show in leads 1, aVL and left sided chest leads. *Posterior wall* infarction is less common and often more difficult to recognise. As none of the chest "V" leads face the posterior wall of the heart, diagnosis must be made from the reciprocal changes that are especially seen in leads V1, V2 and aVF.

> Whenever characteristic changes are seen on the ECG, always look for reciprocal changes on the leads in opposite polarity to those facing the area of infarct

FIGURE 41

The leads that face the area of infarct will show S–T elevations

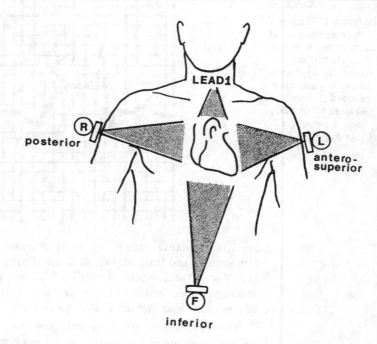

Figure 41 illustrates how limb lead 1 and the anterior chest leads both face the anterior and superior surface of the heart whilst the leads aVF, 2 and 3 face the inferior surface.

There are of course other anatomical and conduction abnormalities of the heart that will produce Q wave changes and the student must be aware that not all Q waves of over 25 % amplitude are related to myocardial infarction, e.g. idiopathic hypertrophic sub-aortic stenosis (IHSS) will show deep Q waves that are due to the thickening of the ventricular septum. It takes longer to penetrate and depolarise the septum, hence wider Q waves will occur.

The criteria for assessing myocardial infarction are not well defined, although it should be remembered that the appearance of

FIGURE 42

Typical 12 lead
electrocardiogram of an
anterior wall infarction.
Note the S–T elevation
in the anterior chest
leads.

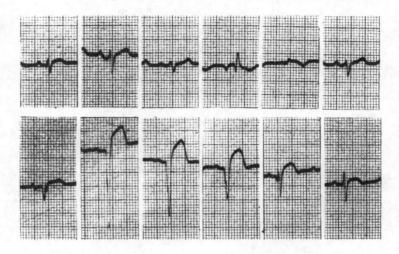

a pathological Q wave in any one lead should be ignored. This rule applies especially to the leads 3, aVR and V1. There is much more support of a diagnosis if the Q waves are accompanied by changes in the S–T segment and/or T wave, although here again there is an exception: often in the presence of a restricted infarct that involves the subendocardial layer of the ventricles there are S–T and T wave changes *without* abnormal Q waves!

2 *The Monitored Patient*

Oscilloscopic or video monitors are used in many areas of the modern hospital for the visualisation of numerous physiological functions that may be presented in either analog or digital format or both. The instrument may be power or battery operated or a combination of both, having its controls located on the fascia that will enable the operator to obtain a satisfactory presentation of the monitored event.

In the field of cardiology, monitors are frequently used in conjunction with other specialised equipment, such as multi-channel physiological cath lab recorders, CCU computers, Holter analysers, EST equipment, pacemaker analysers, echocardiograph machines, etc.

GENERAL CONCEPTS

They may be *single, dual* or *multi-channel* depending on specific requirements. A cath lab monitor is likely to be ceiling-suspended and slaved from a physiological recorder allowing eight or more channels to be presented, especially if *electrophysiological studies (EPS)* are performed. A CCU monitor may require 3–4 channels whereas a Holter monitor may have two or more channels. For pacemaker analyses and programming, a single channel may suffice.

The requirements of the simple form of a cardiac monitor are similar for all types irrespective of the manufacturer. It will have:

❏ an input socket that will accept a patient cable or any physiological transducer to be connected;

❏ a position or centering control that will allow the operator to adjust the function centrally on the screen (unless this be done automatically or the monitor has a fixed baseline);

❏ a sensitivity or gain control that will allow the amplitude of the displayed signal to be increased or decreased;

❏ upper and lower alarm controls that will provide audible and/or visual alarms to be triggered should the function increase or decrease beyond preset limits.

A number of the older type of cardiac monitors that interrogate a single ECG lead using a three wire cable are still used in many hospitals. They record the ECG lead commonly known as a *"Cm lead"* or chest monitor lead. This is a bipolar lead that records the potential difference between two active electrodes that are located on the anterior surface of the chest wall. Connection of each of these electrodes is via colour coded cables that have polarity in relation to one another, i.e. one is negative, usually white and the other positive, usually black. A third "ground" electrode coloured green is also attached to the chest wall serving no purpose other than to maintain the patient at ground level. Many monitors of European origin have colour codes of red (negative), yellow (positive) and black (ground). Some monitors may also be isolated from ground using three active electrodes.

Obtaining the ECG In order to obtain a good quality electrocardiogram from a monitor it is essential that four conditions are met:

❑ There must be good electrical conduction at the skin/electrode interface.

❑ The electrode must have good adhesive properties.

❑ The contact between the electrode and cable must be secure.

❑ The ECG from the patient should be large in amplitude and artefact free.

The first of these qualities is found in most silver/silver chloride electrodes. The operator should ensure that after removal of the electrode from its package that the sponge pad is moist and that the gel has not dried. Dried or partially dried electrodes may create gross movement artefact or the absence of an ECG tracing on the monitor.

The second quality means that the adhesive property of the electrode must be sound. Electrodes that have been stored for long periods or have been subjected to heat may lose their adhesive qualities.

Before applying a disposable electrode to the skin it is essential that all hair over the site be removed and the area be cleaned with a cotton swab lightly soaked in ether. This highly volatile substance is preferred to alcohol since it more readily removes the fat and skin moisture. If an alcohol swab is used the alcohol must be allowed to evaporate completely before the electrode is applied, otherwise the adhesiveness of the electrode will be destroyed. The electrode backing should then be removed and the electrode applied to the skin with firm pressure to its surrounds.

The third quality, namely a reliable electrode/cable contact is assured by a distinct "snap" of the female cable connector when affixed to its male electrode counterpart. If the spring-loaded type of connector is used make sure it has not lost its tension.

A suitably derived ECG depends on electrode siting and the technologist should be aware that *within limits*, the further apart the active electrodes are located on the patient's chest the larger will be the amplitude of the ECG signal. It must also be remembered that the amplitude of the ECG will be governed by the location of the two active electrodes on the patient's chest and the pathology present. Certain diseases may produce low amplitude signals or a change in the frontal electrical axis of the heart. A deviation of the normal axis is often seen in tall thin or short obese patients and commonly seen in pregnancy.

Application of the electrodes

Many of the problems associated with ECG monitoring are due to the poor application or siting of electrodes.

Except when recording multiple leads which are placed on specific positions on the torso, it is obviously technically better to generate a large ECG signal from the patient, by a suitable choice of electrode placement. Small ECG complexes will require maximal adjustment of the sensitivity or gain control of the monitor in order to obtain an 'interpretable' ECG. Not only will the ECG be unnecessarily magnified but so will movement artefacts, muscle tremor and superimposed alternating current interference.

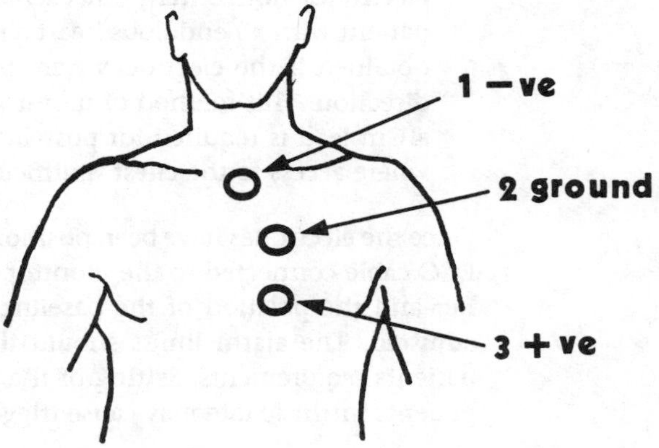

FIGURE 43
Recommended electrode sites when using a three lead monitoring system

1 − ve

2 ground

3 + ve

There are two simple methods by which a large ECG signal may be obtained from the two active chest electrodes:

1. Study the V leads of the patient's 12 lead diagnostic electrocardiogram. Which has the largest QRS amplitude? If the heart has a normal frontal axis this is usually V2 i.e. the fourth intercostal space left of the sternum.

   Position one electrode at this site and connect the positive (black) electrode cable to it.

Position a second electrode to the right of the flat superior portion of the sternum and connect the negative (white) electrode cable to it.

A third electrode (green) may be positioned between the two, and although its site is not of importance it does allow the electrode cable to remain in-line and thus avoid any possible entanglement of the cables during sleeping.

This method has the disadvantage of partially obliterating the area conventionally reserved for placement of a defibrillator paddle. It also does not permit the ECG V2 to be used for diagnostic recording. However, the advantages of having a near perfect ECG recording on the cardiac monitor may be considered to outweigh these inconveniences. When defibrillation is required the defib paddle may be positioned to the right of the upper Cm electrode. When recording a 12 lead diagnostic electrocardiogram the V2 suction electrode may be placed inferior to the lower Cm electrode. (NB It is important to make note of this inferior position of V2 on the recording).

2. The second method involves positioning the active electrodes in-line with the electrical axis of the heart. In the obese patient with a "horizontal" heart this might necessitate applying the electrodes horizontally on each side of the chest wall. In a patient with a pendulous heart a more acceptable ECG may be obtained if the electrodes were positioned in a more vertical direction. This method of monitoring is often necessary when a Cm lead is required for post-surgical monitoring of patients where access to the chest is difficult due to bandaging.

Once the electrodes have been positioned on the chest wall and the ECG cable connected to the monitor, the sensitivity of the amplifier and the position of the baseline of the ECG signal must be adjusted. The alarm limits should then be set according to the patients requirements. Setting of the alarm limits too close to the patients intrinsic rate may cause triggering of false alarms.

On the other hand it is often necessary to closely adjust the limits when monitoring a patient whose heart is controlled by a cardiac pacemaker, whether implanted or externally positioned.

Note: Very few of these simple CRT monitors (and some computer-controlled monitors) are able to distinguish between a captured paced beat, i.e. a pacemaker impulse that is followed by a QRS complex and a pacemaker impulse that is not. It is not difficult to imagine such a monitor registering a heart rate that is triggered by the pacemaker spike alone whilst the patient has ventricular standstill.

Persistent AC interference

Alternating current (AC) interferences are the mains frequency oscillations that are superimposed upon the electrocardiogram baseline. Its presence may signify an electrical current pathway through the patient.

If, after correct placement of the electrodes, alternating current interference is seen superimposed on the monitored ECG (as regular oscillations of the baseline), the following checks should be made:

❑ Electrodes dried out. i.e. no gel.
❑ Poor skin preparation.
❑ Poor contact between electrode and cable.
❑ Open circuit cable.
❑ An unearthed power plug of the monitor or of any other electrically operated apparatus e.g. bed, infuser, etc.
❑ Patient in close proximity to other electrical appliances, i.e. fluorescent lighting tubes, electric motors, diathermy apparatus, etc.
❑ Faulty monitor.

There is *always* a reason why AC interference is present on an ECG monitor. It may indicate that the patient is electrically live in respect to ground, which may under certain circumstances be a potentially harmful situation!

Multi-lead monitors

In areas where ECG monitoring of the critical ill patient is required it has been shown that simultaneous monitoring and analysis of two or more leads is preferred.[5] It is likely that one lead monitoring may prevent the detection of minute changes of the S–T segment, P wave direction, QRS axes and the ability to differentiate between VT and SVT etc. With the aid of computer processing the detection and diagnoses of arrhythmias and S–T segment deviations can be more accurately performed. Two or more leads prevent loss of monitoring, and interpretation, in the presence of one lead failure.

Computer-aided monitors

Today, many physiological monitors operate with the aid of a computer, with either monochrome or colour video systems, which will allow many functions to be visualised and calculations made.

Most operate in conjunction with specific *modules*, that are fitted into adjacent slide compartments. These modules are used for the detection, amplification and control of distinct physiological functions, such as the electrocardiogram, invasive pressure, non-invasive blood pressure, temperature, cardiac output, O_2 saturation, arrhythmia, respiration, etc, and control the output of the various sensors and transducers required to measure each parameter. Non-modular monitors may have parameters contained within the computer software program, in which case the required parameter to be measured and monitored would have to be manually created from the keyboard or monitor controls.

In no area of the modern hospital is high level arrhythmia and S–T analysis more important than in the Coronary Care Unit. These facilities are of special importance when rhythm disturbances are of major concern, and their detection within limits, accurately presented. The way this is achieved is controlled by an *algorithm*, another name for the set of instructions that the computer is given to carry out its required task. These instructions allow the computer to (a) recognise and digitally sample a suitable incoming signal, (b) filter it to remove baseline artefact and noise, and then (c) pattern classify the QRS into various forms of ectopy or ventricular rhythms. It does this by first recognising a series of beats as being 'normal' in regard to the morphology and timing for that particular patient. The final pattern or *template* of the QRS complex contained within the series is stored in memory for subsequent comparison with future QRS complexes. At the same time the computer recognises the interval between each 'normal' QRS complex. Any deviation of the stored shape or timing interval, as compared to the normal template is at once recognised as an arrhythmia.

FIGURE 44

The computer process of interpretation of the incoming electrocardiogram

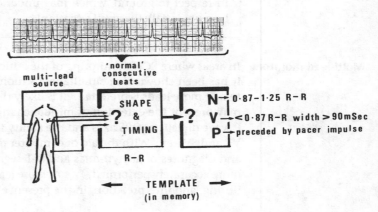

The computer may then arrange the QRS complex into either *normal, paced, ventricular, supraventricular,* or *ectopic*. It detects a normal beat by the R–R interval; a paced beat as one that is preceded by a pacer impulse, and a ventricular beat, by the QRS width and R–R interval. It will also detect any missed beats and artefacts. Analysing with the use of a computer allows more reliable assessment of such arrhythmias and aberrations as:

❏ asystole
❏ bigeminy

- bradycardia
- couplets
- pauses
- premature ventricular contractions
- irregular beats
- R on T
- tachycardia
- ventricular fibrillation, and
- pacemaker artefacts.

Each of the above aberrations must meet specific criteria in order that the computer may recognise them. For example, couplets would be recognised by the appearance of four consecutive beats, the first and last as normal and the second and third as ventricular (NVVN).

The greater the number of leads analysed by the monitor the more accurate the interpretation. Technology does not yet allow absolute reliable analysis of atrial events other than the effects they may have on ventricular rhythms. Often P waves are superimposed on QRS and T waves and are therefore difficult to be recognised by the computer. One method[6] involves sampling the arrhythmia, averaging the QRS–T complex contained within the sample and then subtracting this from the arrhythmia sample, leaving only the P waves. These P waves would then be timed and related to the original QRS complexes of the arrhythmia sample. Such arrhythmias as A–V dissociation, retrograde atrial conduction, junctional rhythm, and SVT would be more accurately interrogated.

The analysis of S–T segment deviations is sometimes questionable as is dual chamber pacing analysis, especially when related to 'non-capture' and 'non-sense' situations. One should realise that often the computer cannot compete with the interpretive skills of an expert electro-cardiologist but is does allow one to overview stored information, correct inaccuracies and store and retrieve information far more efficiently.

The minor drawbacks with some modern computerised monitors is that a large part of the screen is taken up with digital data, and few permit the physiological parameters to be amplified sufficiently to view and interpret from distances greater than from the immediate bedside. This may not be problematical if monitoring is performed at a central console.

Some are not user-friendly and are often underutilised. In a busy coronary care or post-surgical cardiac unit much time may be spent by nursing personnel distracted by the array of numerous controls, often at the expense of patient care. However, once staff are adequately trained they do provide information that cannot be obtained by single lead monitors.

An important advantage of computer-aided monitors is that they are able to perform many functions, such as storage and retrieval of data, produce graphs and calculations, supply 24 hour Holter recordings, allow sorting of any recorded parameter and, when used in a *local area network (LAN)* are able to communicate with any other monitor attached to the network.

Requirements There are certain general technical requirements that should be considered when acquiring a cardiac monitor:

❑ Is the monitor isolated from the patient? This means that under no circumstances can electrical currents be transmitted to the patient from the monitor via the ECG cable and electrodes.

❑ Is the monitor protected from overload voltages in excess of 5000 volts and will the baseline return to its normal position within seconds after the administration of a defibrillatory shock?

❑ If the monitor is to be used in the presence of cautery or other high frequency emitting devices, will it allow continual visualisation of the ECG?

❑ Is there adequate filtration to prevent electrical noise interference? How does it cope with alternating interference from power sources?

❑ Does the monitor detect QRS complexes of low amplitude? If a multi-lead analysis system is used this should not be a problem. If a single channel monitor is used, will the QRS be detected should the patients axis be changed when, for example, he turns in his bed?

❑ Is the time base of the CRT or video accurate? (This refers to the sweep of the trace as it traverses across the screen).

❑ Do the alarms respond accurately to arrhythmias that are life threatening?

❑ Is the monitor "user friendly"? i.e. simple to use without causing too much hesitation?

❑ Are the traces clearly displayed?

If a computer-based monitoring system is used with a data management system, further questions may be asked:

❑ Has it the ability to detect pacemaker discharge and to recognise non-capture, the condition when there is no QRS following the pacemaker spike?

❑ Are the S–T measurement points fixed or can they be manually manipulated?

❑ Which arrhythmias is the monitor able to recognise and can they be classified?

❏ How dependent is the monitor on a central station to function effectively? Will a power loss at the central station cause loss of information?

❏ Is it able to detect and record the onset and offset of tachycardias?

❏ Is it able to ignore the presence of repeatable VPB's that would overload the storage system?

These points may not all be of particular importance to general ICU care, but are often relevant in the *Coronary Care Unit (CCU)*.

HAEMODYNAMIC MONITORING

Haemodynamic monitoring by means of a balloon tipped flow directed catheter inserted percutaneously via one of the accessible large veins (anterior cubital, internal jugular, subclavian) has become an accepted practice in the management of the critically ill patient. Prior to this technique, much reliance was placed on central venous pressure monitoring to assess cardiopulmonary distress. The Swan–Ganz technique allows continuous monitoring of pulmonary artery and intermittent pulmonary capillary wedge pressures which specifically reflects left atrial pressure. Normally, the atrial pressure curve closely resembles the ventricular diastolic waveform (except during the isovolumetric contraction period) and as this approximates the ventricular end diastolic pressure (LVEDP), ventricular dysfunction may be determined.

The catheter The most commonly used catheter is the 7F thermodilution type consisting of 3 lumen:

❏ Lumen 1 terminates at the tip of the catheter.
❏ Lumen 2 terminates 30 cm proximally from the tip.
❏ Lumen 3 terminates within the balloon positioned at the tip.

The thermistor element used to measure intravascular temperature is located 4 cm proximally from the tip. (q.v. Section 2 Cardiac Output)

Catheter placement In its correct position the tip should lie in the distal portion of the left or right pulmonary artery.

Lumen 1 is used to measure *pulmonary artery pressure (PAP)* and/ or to withdraw mixed venous blood samples (with the balloon deflated), and pulmonary capillary wedge pressure (with the balloon inflated).

The Proximal Lumen 2 should lie within the right atrium and is used to measure central venous pressure or to infuse intravenous fluids, or to inject fluids for cardiac output determinations.

The Balloon Lumen 3 opens 10 mm from the tip within the balloon. The diameter of the balloon is approximately 13 mm when fully inflated and surrounds and protrudes over the tip but does not, under normal circumstances, occlude the distal lumen.

Indications for use

□ Acute myocardial infarction — to determine left ventricular function as a guide to fluid requirements, particularly in the hypotensive patient.

□ Pre-operative management of compromised cardiovascular function.

□ Acute and chronic congestive heart failure, especially when sodium nitroprusside is used.

□ Determination at the bedside of cardiac output in order to assess the effects of drug therapy.

□ Trauma and burn injuries requiring the use of large intravenous fluid volumes especially when left ventricular function is compromised.

Technique

The procedure should only be performed by an experienced physician accompanied by a nurse familiar with the technique. ECG and pressure monitoring is essential and operators should be aware of the complications that may be encountered during and after introduction of the catheter.

The most common approach of introduction is via direct subclavian puncture although the internal jugular approach is sometimes preferred.

The patient should lie flat on his back with the neck extended. Before introduction the balloon integrity must be checked by submerging the tip in sterile saline and inflating it. Catheter lumen 1 and 2 should be flushed with Heparin solution. The flow-directed catheter should be introduced with care, and kinking prior and during insertion avoided. Handling of the area of the catheter where the thermistor is located must be avoided at all times.

After adjustment of the transducer zero to mid chest level the distal lumen is attached to the pressure transducer and the pressure monitored. The catheter is then advanced under pressure guidance until a right atrial waveform is seen. The balloon is then inflated and the catheter deliberately advanced until it reaches the pulmonary artery, as determined by the pressure waveform. During advancement to the pulmonary artery a right ventricular waveform should be observed on the monitor.

Once the catheter is located in the pulmonary artery, the balloon is deflated and further slowly advanced until a wedge pressure is seen. The catheter is then withdrawn approximately 2–4 cm where it should then be located in its proper position in a distal pulmonary artery. The balloon is then inflated in order to obtain a wedged capillary pressure.

It is important that when inflating the balloon, pressure applied to the plunger of the syringe should be done *slowly* and halted as soon as the PCWP is seen. Should a change of resistance be felt, inflation should cease at that point. "Wedging" of the catheter once the balloon is inflated will invariably result in a waveform of small pulse pressure having minor oscillations corresponding with respiration. However, in the presence of pulmonary disease the pulmonary wedge pressure may fluctuate markedly with respiration. In such a condition wedge pressure should be measured during the phase of end expiration — the point at which the left atrial pressure most closely correlates.

Once the balloon is deflated these respiratory oscillations should not be pronounced and a pulmonary arterial waveform be seen. An arterial waveform with large respiratory oscillations usually indicates a distal siting of the catheter.

Should a wedge waveform exist when the balloon is deflated the catheter is too distal and should be withdrawn immediately to avoid possible thrombus formation at its tip and/or infarction.

Normal pressure ranges (mm Hg)

Right atrium (RA)	0–7	mean 0–5
Right ventricle (RV)	22–30/0–5	end diastolic 0–8
Pulmonary artery (PA)	15–30/5–15	mean 10 / 20
Pulmonary Capillary wedge	(PCWP)	mean 6 – 12

Pressure interpretation Increased pulmonary wedge pressure indicates an increase in left atrial pressure and, in absence of mitral valve disease, an elevated end-diastolic pressure denoting left ventricular dysfunction (resulting in decreased cardiac output).

Decreased pulmonary wedge pressure indicates a decrease in left ventricular end-diastolic pressure resulting in reduced cardiac output due to hypovolaemia.

An acute rise in pulmonary artery pressure with a normal wedge pressure suggests a primary pulmonary disorder e.g. pulmonary embolus.

An *increase* in both pulmonary artery and wedge pressures suggests a primary cardiac disorder e.g. Left Ventricular Failure.

Positive end-expiratory pressure (PEEP) may influence wedge pressure measurement and its correlation with pulmonary artery and left ventricular end-diastolic pressures. Peep pressures of greater than 5 cm during the negative pressure phase may increase wedge pressure (due to inhibition of ventricular return from the pulmonary vascular bed) and decrease cardiac output. A good approximation of the real pulmonary capillary wedge pressure (PCWP) may be obtained by subtracting the intrathoracic pressure from the measured pressure.

Conditions in which PCWP may be higher than left ventricular end-diastolic pressure:

- ❑ Mitral stenosis.
- ❑ Mitral valve prolapse with incompetence.
- ❑ Left atrial myxoma.
- ❑ Pulmonary Venous obstruction.
- ❑ High intra-alveolar pressure (continuous positive pressure ventilation).

REMEMBER

- ❑ Acute mitral insufficiency will often produce a large "v" wave on the PCWP recording that may obscure the "a" wave and cause difficulty in its interpretation.
- ❑ Most forms of restrictive and constrictive heart disease will often produce what may appear equal diastolic pressures of the right ventricle and pulmonary artery.
- ❑ When unexpectedly high PCWP is measured, the catheter should be withdrawn and repositioned in another site.
- ❑ PCWP can *never* be higher than the PAEDP!

Conditions in which PCWP pressure may be lower than left ventricular end-diastolic pressure (LVEDP):

- ❑ Stiff left ventricle.
- ❑ High left ventricular end-diastolic pressure (> 25 mm Hg).

REMEMBER

Since there is normally no obstruction between the occluded segment of the pulmonary artery and the left atrium, the pressure recorded by the distal catheter lumen will, for all practical purposes, be identical to the left atrial pressure. Within the range of approximately 6–20 mm Hg this pressure is virtually the same as the left ventricular end diastolic pressure..

The one condition in which the right ventricular end-diastolic pressure may exceed the wedge pulmonary capillary pressure is right ventricular infarction

Technical considerations

In order for the catheter to "float" to its destination, aided by an inflated balloon at its distal tip, it must of necessity be manufactured of a compliant material. Inevitably, this does reduce the undamped natural frequency of the catheter. It is for this reason that French sizes below 7 should, if possible, be avoided.

Complications during introduction of catheter

- Pneumothorax: a comparatively high incidence of pneumothorax associated with direct subclavian insertion and subsequent accidental injection of air into the pleural space is reported.
- Thrombophlebitis
- Haemorrhaging at insertion site.
- Air embolism due to inadequate flushing of pressure lines
- Ruptured chordae — a rare complication
- Knotting of catheter — a rare complication usually avoidable
- Ventricular tachycardia / fibrillation

Later complications

- Arrhythmias due to migration of catheter across the pulmonary valve.
- Pulmonary Artery Perforation or rupture usually caused by overinflation of balloon.
- Pulmonary infarction or haemorrhage, due to prolonged wedging of catheter, thrombus formation or migration of catheter into a small branch of artery.
- Tricuspid and/or pulmonary valve damage
- Balloon Rupture. When the catheter is in the correct position and (a) no wedge pressur is obtained and (b) the balloon offers no resistance when inflated, then rupture should be suspected. Do not inflate further.
- Infection. This incidence is high in the elderly.

Care must be taken to ensure that all pressure transducers, tubing and taps are sterile prior to use.

Whilst many studies have shown haemodynamic monitoring using a pulmonary artery catheter as being clinically beneficial in patients with acute myocardial infarction,[7, 8] there is no doubt that the introduction of a PA catheter does often subject the patient to unnecessary risk due to the high incidence of complications.[9, 10] Others have shown there to be no therapeutic benefit to those patients with acute MI that are complicated by congestive heart failure, hypotension or cardiogenic shock.[11]

RECORDING TECHNIQUES

The accuracy of any recorded event, whether it be a pressure pulse, an electrocardiogram or other physiological phenomenon is as important to the patient as the interpretation made by the physician, and unless the apparatus on which the event is recorded is technically sound, it would be unwise and morally wrong to draw any conclusions with regard to abnormalities. Firstly let us consider the recording of the electrocardiogram, the most frequently monitored and recorded of all physiological functions.

It is assumed that the reader is familiar with the technique of recording, including the application of electrodes to the patient.

Today, many different types of ECG machines are commercially available that vary in their methods of recording, format of presentation, storage and interpretation. Basically all have certain features in common. They:

❑ amplify an alternating electrical signal of approximately 1 millivolt (the ECG).

❑ block the direct current signal of approximately 30 mV or more, on which the ECG is superimposed, commonly known as the "skin potential".

❑ record the final electrocardiogram on paper.

Some will allow either a manual or automatic presentation of the order in which the leads are recorded. This may be in 4 groups of three, 2 groups of six or as 1 group of 12, or any other format.

Amplification of the alternating current (AC) ECG signal would be electronically simple were it not for the fact that it is superimposed upon a comparatively high direct current (DC) level. Both are of variable amplitude, one dependent upon lead selection and cardiac abnormality and the other influenced by skin impedance. Whenever an ECG lead position is changed, not only does the ECG morphology alter but also the level of the DC component. For example, the ECG from lead 2 may be superimposed upon a DC level of 200 mV whilst it may be upon 20 mV in lead 1. It is because of this high DC component that either (a) an AC coupled preamplifier and signal amplifier or (b) a direct current restoration circuit is required to block the DC level. The capacitance-coupled preamplifier blocks the DC component allowing only the AC electrocardiographic component to be further amplified, whilst in the restoration circuit the signal undergoes a digital transformation that is modulated and demodulated before the signal is finally recorded.

Using such a "feedback" circuit, the low frequency response would be zero. The high frequency response may be as high as 200 Hz although most ECG machines have response characteristics within the range of 0 (or 0.05) to 100 Hz.

FIGURE 45

The input potentials of the AC coupled electrocardiograph

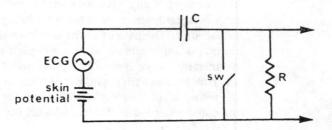

Figure 45 illustrates how the ECG signal, which may be imagined as an alternating generator whose output is superimposed on a direct current voltage of some 30 times its value, is processed by an *AC coupled pre-amplifier*. The capacitor C in the circuit permits the alternating ECG component to pass whilst blocking the DC component. It charges to a level equal to the value of the skin potential of the patient.

Because of the varying values of the DC component, the charge on C will also vary, which when subsequently amplified, would cause gross drift of the recording mechanism. To overcome this problem a "blocking" switch SW allows the capacitor C to be charged directly from its source instead of via resistor R, so that a new value of charge may be quickly attained. The modern electrocardiograph performs this task automatically whenever a change of lead or new format of leads are recorded.

There are a number of ways in which physiological events may be recorded. The mechanism may be a plotter that operates on both X and Y axes, in which case the ECG signal is first processed by the input amplifier, then digitized by an A-D (analog-digital) converter before it is temporarily stored in memory. It is then able to be recorded by a single pen in multichannel formats.

FIGURE 46

The four elements of the Hewlett Packard Pagewriter Cardiograph. The input isolates the DC signal, has electrical safety features and converts the waveform into a digital signal. The digitized signals are passed into memory where the data is stored before recorded.

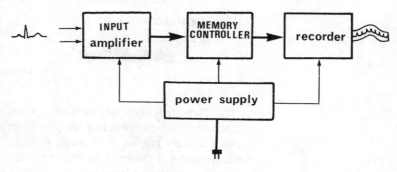

A commonly used recording mechanism is the direct current *D'Arsonval galvanometer*, in which a rectangular coil, pivoted between the poles of a magnet, reacts within a magnetic field, producing a torque. The degree through which the coil rotates is a direct measurement of the current flowing through the coil and the deflection is observed by movement of a pointer or stylus attached to the coil. Methods of recording utilising the D'Arsonval galvanometer may be in the form of a fine tube, through which ink under high pressure is allowed to spray as a jet on paper; or the stylus tip may be electrically heated and made to contact a prepared wax paper on which a black impression is made.

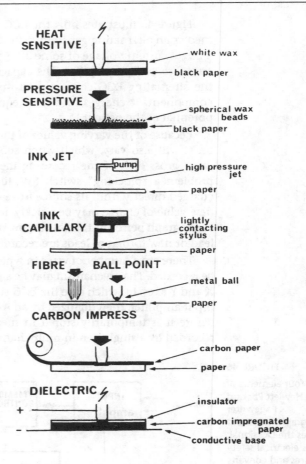

FIGURE 47

Various recording methods

The *Thermal Array printer* as used in most modern electrocardiographs and physiological recording systems consists of a series of resistive heaters known as thermal elements. Many hundreds of these elements positioned in-line form the printhead, the heat from which allows an image to be formed onto a thermoreactive paper. In order to drive such a printer mechanism a computer processor is essential. The main function of the *central processing unit (CPU)* is to control the incoming and outgoing data to the printer, control the printer memory *(RAM)* (q.v. Glossary) the paper speed, the temperature of the printhead and to provide an interface to the printer.

For the ECG machine, or any physiological recording apparatus for that matter, to faithfully present the electrical pattern emitted by the heart, it must possess certain qualities:

❑ Linearity
❑ Stability

❏ Zero balance
❏ Adequate frequency response.

The following tests will enable the operator to check some of these parameters. Much depends of the type of recorder. Most microprocessor controlled machines that have a DC restoration input and/or convert the incoming analogue signal to a digital format, may not allow manual manipulation of other than the bare minimum of controls, whilst many of the older physiological multichannel recording systems do allow operator access.

Linearity The word "linear" describes the relation between two varying quantities when one varies in direct proportion to the other, so that a graphic presentation would produce a straight line. Two important variables are voltage and stylus excursion. If a given voltage of x units causes the stylus to deflect y centimetres, each incremental increase or decrease of voltage should produce a proportional increase or decrease of pen excursion over the entire paper recording width, (dx = dy).

Study of the linear response pattern will determine (a) whether the recorder waveform will be accurately reproduced in amplitude over the entire recording range and (b) the extent to which the stylus can traverse without cutting off the signal.

FIGURE 48
Checks of:
(a) Linearity,
(b) Sensitivity and
(c) deflection

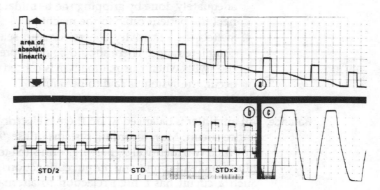

Check as follows:

1. Adjust the stylus to the centre of the recording paper and accurately calibrate for a deflection of 1 cm. with the 1mV source.
2. Run paper drive at 25mm/sec speed with one hand controlling the stylus centering knob.
3. Adjust stylus to a position 1 cm from the top edge of the recording span and inject 1mV signals at 5 mm levels, simultaneously deflecting the stylus towards the bottom edge.
4. Study of the amplitude of each square wave will reveal any alinearity present as each initial square wave rise should be 1cm

in amplitude (Figure 48a). Cut-off appearing at the extreme edges of the paper chart will indicate a non-linear area. Effective linear excursion can only be guaranteed between any two adjacent wave forms of equal amplitude.

5. Check should also be made to ascertain the linearity of the signal deflection. Adjust the stylus to deflect exactly 2 cm/mV on the double sensitivity setting, and then switch to normal and half sensitivity settings at the same time injecting a 1 mV signal on each position. The amplitude of the calibration 1 mV signals should be successively halved (Figure 48b).

6. Reset the sensitivity to normal 1 cm/mV and deflect the stylus over the entire paper width. There should be no electrical or mechanical cut-off of the stylus within the recording range (figure 48c).

Stability This refers to the movement of the stylus under conditions of zero input, and may be checked as follows:

1. Set lead selector to STD or CAL position.

2. Turn sensitivity control to maximum and adjust stylus to centre of paper.

3. Using a conductive terminal bar, short circuit the pins of the amplifier input, or the pins of the patient cable. (This may be adequately done by gripping the terminal pins in a vice). Connect the patient cable to the machine.

4. Switch the sensitivity control or lead selector throughout its complete range. There should be no appreciable movement of the stylus when this manoeuvre is carried out. Should no drift occur, the system is said to be stable.

Balance An amplifier is balanced when there is electrical equilibrium in the entire circuit. Most recording systems utilise "balanced" amplifiers in which two identical signals are connected to operate in opposite phase and with input and output connections balanced to ground. Such a circuit has a high rejection to alternating and unwanted currents. Out of balance is often caused by component ageing which may be easily adjusted by the operator or service contractor.

Test as follows:

1. With selector switch on STD or CAL position, adjust sensitivity to minimum position.

2. Adjust stylus to centre of paper.

3. Rotate or switch sens.tivity control to its maximum position and return to its minimum position. Record changes.

There should be a minimal change of stylus deflection during this procedure.

FIGURE 49

Balance check showing minimum and maximum settings of sensitivity control

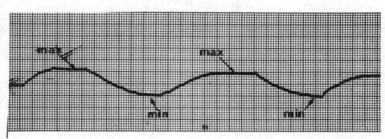

Frequency response

This refers to the variation of frequency to the gain or loss of signal amplitude and may be considered as a measurement of the recording sensitivity to various applied frequencies. It is obvious that any system of oscillation is limited to a maximum frequency, depending upon its mass and inertia. The less the mass the higher is the frequency at which the system will oscillate and conversely, the higher the mass the lower the frequency. For example, if a sinusoidal current of constant amplitude is applied to the input of an amplifier and the frequency of current increased from say zero to 500 hertz, because of the mass of the stylus, a point would be reached where the galvanometer would no longer respond to such rapid vibrations in a linear fashion. In other words its amplitude would decrease and continue to do so until it reached zero movement. The frequency at which the stylus begins to decrease is generally referred to as its *FLAT RESPONSE;* in other words the amplitude is constant up to that point. The term 'flat' is purely relative and in engineering practice, a frequency of 100 Hz would have a response of 70.7 %, it being the value of $\frac{1}{\sqrt{2}}$ of the maximum value, i.e. 3 db down, commonly termed the cut-off frequency.

FIGURE 50

The frequency response of a recorder illustrating the decrease of signal amplitude after application of a sine wave to the input varying between 10 and 100 Hz

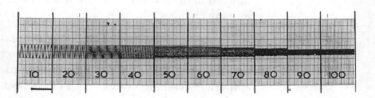

It is believed that frequencies of over 2000 Hz are contained in the human electrocardiogram and Langer[12] has suggested that the ECG recorder should have a frequency response of 330 Hz and probably much higher to faithfully record the electrocardiogram.

Some, however, believe that 200 Hz is a minimum flat frequency requirement.[13, 14]

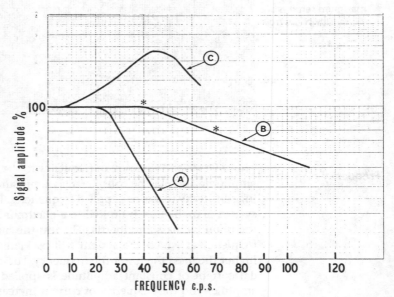

Although many present day electrocardiographs have a flat response within 3dB from 0 to 100 Hz with automatic calibration and stabilizing facilities, it has been shown that QRS amplitude errors greater than 50 micro volts can occur in over 10 % of adult recordings when this frequency bandwidth is used. Higher upper frequency limits are now generally accepted. However, as it is not usually convenient to check the response of an ECG machine, or any other physiological recording system that uses a blocking capacitor to supress the DC level, with a signal generator, study of the simple calibration square wave will give the operator a good indication of how the machine will respond to both slow and fast moving changes.

Figure 52 illustrates the three degrees of damping of the square wave when testing the response of a physiological recorder. In the upper tracing the 1mV signal is applied to the recorder and the amplitude calibrated to exactly 1 cm deflection of the stylus. The left-hand wave shows a moderate overdamped response that is characterised by the roundness of the corners and slow rise time of the deflection. Such a response would give rise to a roundness of the ECG waveform and slurring of its high frequency components.

The middle recording is the ideal which has a fast rise time, completely 'square' corners and flat right-angled top and bottom.

The rise time indicates that the high response is adequate, and the flat portions that the low response is acceptable.

The extreme case of underdamping as shown in the upper right hand recording is presented by a large overshoot of the stylus. This condition would cause the fast moving QRS components of the ECG to be grossly exaggerated.

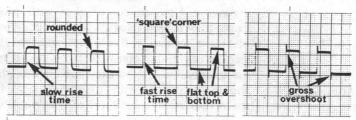

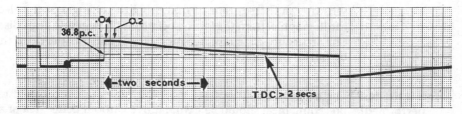

Time decay constant (TDC) This is the time required for an electrical quantity to rise to 63.2 % $(1 - 1/e)$ of its final value, or to fall to 36.8 % ($1/e$ where e = the exponential function 2.718) of its initial value. By applying a 1 mV prolonged square wave the operator is able to judge more accurately the lower frequency response of the system. Evaluation is made of the time taken for the curve to decay to a level of 36.8 % of its initial value after depression of the 1mV calibration button. The time decay constant should exceed 2 seconds when applied to the input of an AC preamplfier. The technologist should, however, be aware that many recording systems, especially those with digital automatic recording facilities, do not allow prolongation of the square wave to be measured after depression of the 1 mV button.

EXERCISE STRESS TESTING

Physicians have long known of the dramatic changes that occur to cardiovascular function during exercise as compared to resting conditions. In 1935, Masters[15] formulated an exercise protocol according to the sex, weight and age of the patient that was based on the number of ascents made on a two-sided, two-step wooden platform. The work performed was easily calculated from the product of the height of the step in metres, the rate of stepping per minute and the body weight of the subject in kilograms. Such an inexpensive, simple and effective method was used many years for the objective diagnosis of coronary artery disease that was related to the changes of the ECG (invariably recorded on a single channel ECG machine) shown during exercise.

Today the Masters step test, often referred as the "Masters twostep", is rarely used as a means of exercise testing, having been superseded in exercise laboratories by the treadmill or bicycle ergometer. Used in conjunction with processor aided electro-cardiographic technology, today's exercise machines are more stable, more accurate and more reproducible allowing multiple ECG leads to be simultaneously recorded. Of the two types, the easier to use treadmill is the most favoured, although the stress laboratory should be equipped with an exercise bicycle for those patients who for medical reasons have difficulty in running.

Exercise stress testing, often termed *graded exercise testing,* is a sensitive and safe means of measuring the changes of the electro-cardiograph pattern that are associated with ischemic heart disease. The procedure has a reported mortality of 0.01 %[16] provided that it be carried out under strict supervision and patient selection.

How is the test performed? The patient should fast for at least 2 hours prior to the test, the preceding meal should be light, fat free without coffee, tea or alcohol, and advised not to discontinue medication unless otherwise informed by a physician. He or she should wear appropriate comfortable clothing and sneakers or flat walking shoes. After strict clinical examination the patient is prepared for the test.

1. The position of the electrodes include the conventional chest leads V1–V6 and the four limb leads attached to the upper areas of the limbs.
2. The skin areas should be well cleaned and prepared using an ether swab and, if necessary shaved.
3. Slight abrasion of the areas with fine sandpaper or a dry cotton swab is recommended prior to attachment of the electrodes.
4. Once the electrodes and fly leads are connected, bandaging of the chest is advised to ensure stable and clean recordings. It is essential that only good quality electrodes be used.
5. After connection of the patient cable to the recorder an initial pre-exercise ECG is taken.
6. The patient is then exercised on the treadmill, the speed and grading of which are adjusted according to a specific program that is suitable for that particular patient.

Throughout the whole procedure, the ECG leads 2, aVF and V5 are usually monitored together with periodic blood pressure measurements which, when related to heart rate, give an indication of myocardial oxygen consumption. On completion of the test the 12 lead ECG and blood pressure are recorded and repeated at intervals of 2, 5 and 10 mins thereafter.

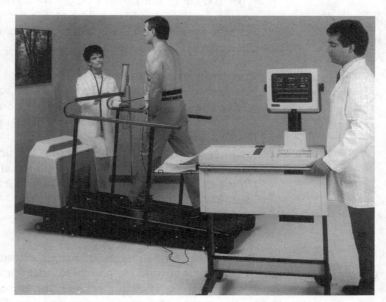

The level of exercise or the *protocol* to which the patient is subjected will depend on his physical and pathological condition. Many physicians use well known and established protocols[17,18,19] or modifications that may suit the exercise capabilities of the patients. The most commonly used are the *BRUCE, NAUGHTON* and *ELLES-TAD* protocols, or modified versions of them.

Below is an example of the Bruce exercise protocol. The first column refers to the time of exercise, the second to the speed of the treadmill and the third to the gradient of the treadmills.

Stage	Time (min)	Speed (miles/h)	(km/h)	Grade (%)
1	3	1.7	2.7	10
2	3	2.5	4.0	12
3	3	3.4	5.5	14
4	3	4.2	6.8	16
5	3	5.0	8.0	18
6	3	5.5	8.8	20
7	3	6.0	9.7	22

<table>
<tr><td>REMEMBER</td><td>Grade or gradient is the amount of slope or inclination as compared to the horizontal of the treadmill. A slope rising 10 cm per 100 cm of horizontal would have a gradient of 10 %. The same gradient would angulate at 6.0 degrees. A gradient of 100 % would have an angulation of 45 degrees.</td></tr>
</table>

The MET   In order to measure and calibrate the amount of exercise achieved by a particular patient it is necessary to use some unit that would relate to the metabolic demands of the body. Such a unit is the MET, or *metabolic equivalent,* a measurement of heat production which in the sitting resting position is equivalent to 50 kilogram calories per square meter of body surface per hour. The unit expressed as oxygen consumption at rest (VO2) approximates $3.5 ml O_2/kg.min$. During exercise of a normal healthy subject levels of over 13, i.e. > 45 ml $O_2/kg.min$ may be reached.

Why is the test performed?

The purpose of the stress test is to attain a heart rate level according to age, that is beyond the normal for that particular patient and to determine the relationship between the amount of work that can be performed and the oxygen consumption. The simple formula of subtracting the age of the patient from the number *220* is used to calculate the *target rate.*

Ideally the patient should be encouraged to exercise to his *maximal effort,* i.e. to a level beyond which any further increase in work *will not* produce any increase in heart rate, blood pressure or oxygen uptake — a point at which myocardial oxygen consumption is at a maximum or near maximum level.

Submaximal testing i.e. exercise to a level of 70 or 85 % of maximum age related heart rate, is often advised when evaluating post myocardial infarction patients, who frequently experience discomfort well before their physiological maximum level.

Predicted maximal heart rates according to age and recommended rate levels for sub-maximal exercise testing.

Age	20	25	30	35	40	45	50	55	60	65	70
max HR	197	195	193	191	189	187	184	182	180	178	176
85 % max	167	166	164	162	161	159	158	155	153	151	148
70 % max	137	136	135	133	132	131	129	127	126	124	123
60 % max	118	117	115	114	113	112	110	109	108	106	105

Note: 85 % = severe, 70 % = moderate, 60 % = mild exercise

Most of the reasons for exercise stress testing are related to the evaluation of the patient with ischemic heart disease and may be performed to:

❑ determine the level of exercise at which ischemic chest pain occurs;

❑ help diagnose the patient with symptoms of *CAD*;

❑ determine the post operative success of those patients having undergone by-pass surgery;

❑ evaluate the patient with high risk factors (familial, obese, smoker, hypertensive etc);

❑ determine the response and subsequent treatment of patients undergoing arrhythmia therapy;

❑ assess cardiac function of those patients with implanted heart valves or pacemakers.

Patient selection   Patients with certain pathological disorders may present too high a risk for exercise stress testing and the importance of evaluation of the patients clinical condition by a physician cannot be too highly stressed. (The high risk disorders mentioned below are not in order of importance).

❑ Ventricular tachyarrhythmias, frequent ectopy especially when multi-focal in origin,2nd or 3rd degree heart block

❑ Unstable angina

❑ Angina at rest

❑ Acute myocardial infarction

❑ Dissecting aneurysm

❑ Known recent embolism

❑ Congestive heart failure

❑ Tight aortic stenosis

There are many other non-cardiac conditions that may cause severe distress to the patient although the risks of some may not outweigh the benefits of the test.

Safety precautions   It should *never* be carried out by one person and a physician must always be in attendance. Emergency resuscitation equipment should be closeby and to include a defibrillator, airways, drugs and if available a transcutaneous pacemaker. The ECG should be continuously monitored and the blood pressure frequently taken throughout the test and for a period of 15 minutes after the test is completed.

Attending personnel should be fully aware of the procedure and know what to do in an emergency situation. They should also be aware of the indications for abortion of the test:

❑ Marked increase in chest pain

❏ Severe discomfort or fatigue
❏ Severe dyspnoea
❏ Dizzyness
❏ Sudden onset of pallor, sweating, mental confusion and/or apprehension.
❏ Any other signs of cardiovascular dysfunction, e.g. a decrease in systolic blood pressure, cyanosis, bradycardia, any ECG aberration that was not present during rest, etc.
❏ When the patient has achieved the maximum heart rate.

What value has the test?

In many studies, exercise stress testing has been well described and proven that a definite correlation exists between positive ECG changes that occur during or after exercise and coronary artery disease.[20,21,22] These changes are usually seen as abnormalities of the S–T segment producing a deviation of greater than 1mm below the baseline.

It is important to remember that:

1. A normal resting ECG does not necessarily indicate the absence of coronary artery disease and the presence of ST–T changes do not necessarily indicate coronary artery disease.[23]
2. The absence of symptoms such as angina, during rest may be provoked during exercise.
3. Other disorders may or may not be related to coronary artery disease, e.g., arrhythmias, dizzyness, respiratory dysfunction, etc.
4. Patients who develop early positive symptoms during the test (angina, ST segment deviation) are at greater risk of early myocardial infarction.
5. The sensitivity of the test is 64 percent which means that 36 percent will not show presence of their coronary artery disease (CAD) when tested, in other words, a negative result will be obtained.

With a predictive value of 80 %, a sensitivity of 64 % and a specificity of 85 %, the investigator should be aware that there are limitations to the accuracy of exercise stress testing.

Choice of equipment

There are many models of EST equipment on the world market and the physician or technologist who is considering purchasing a suitable system for his or her department should first decide how much can be afforded. The barest minimum is the Master two-step used in conjunction with a single channel ECG machine that records the Cm lead 5. Such a system is certainly not recommended to be used in a busy modern exercise stress laboratory where repeatability and accuracy is of utmost importance. In the upper limit are systems that are computer controlled using sophisticated and powerful signal processing techniques that will:

- ❏ allow communication between the recorder and the treadmill.
- ❏ allow the operator to program a set *protocol* of choice (and to modify it at will) that will change the speed and inclination of the treadmill at preprogrammed times.
- ❏ • analyse S–T segment changes from three scalar leads and automatically record.
- ❏ permit storage and retrieval of patient data, selected waveforms and final reports.
- ❏ document and store arrhythmias, and
- ❏ allow the user to change the measurement points, i.e. the isoelectric and J points and the ST levels to suite his requirements, and to program to any desired degree of analysis and report content.

In the mid range are reliable systems that will operate with a standard three channel ECG machine in combination with an electrically operated treadmill or with an exercise bicycle.

Automatic blood pressure devices are often used during tests but do tend to give erroneous readings during the exercise phase. Between the two extremes are many reliable systems using standard three channel ECG machines and an exercise bicycle or treadmill.

Before considering an exercise electrocardiography system the technologist is advised to ask:

- ❏ How good is the recorded ECG? Has the recorder adequate frequency response to (a) eliminate unwanted interference and (b) to reliably distinguish abnormal S–T segmental changes? These two qualities should not be opposed.
- ❏ By what method is the S–T segment measured? Can the isoelectric and J points be adjusted by the operator?
- ❏ What protocols can be accepted? Can these be modified by the operator?
- ❏ Is a final report printed? If so, in what format?
- ❏ Has the ECG monitor a digital heart rate indicator? The generator should not have to record a strip of paper in order to check heart rate!
- ❏ Is the recorder simple to use?
- ❏ Is the treadmill quiet? A noisy treadmill can affect the apprehensiveness of the patient, especially if he or she requires to notify the operator of discomfort during the test.
- ❏ Is the floor of the treadmill safe and will not become slippery when worn?
- ❏ Does the speed of the treadmill operate from zero?
- ❏ Does the treadmill require three-phase wiring? This may not be available in the vicinity of the EST room.

Further reading

❏ Exercise testing and training of individuals with heart disease or at high risk for its development: A handbook for Physicians. *Am. Heart Assn.*, Committee on exercise. 1975.

❏ Fox K, Ilsley C. *The essentials of exercise electrocardiography.* London, Current Med. Literature. 1984.

❏ Ottison D. Graded exercise testing, in Bronson L, (ed): *Textbook of cardiovascular technology.* J.B. Lippincott Company, Philadelphia. 1987.

HIGH RESOLUTION ELECTROCARDIOGRAPHY

The twelve electrocardiographic leads that are presented when a diagnostic ECG is recorded provides much information of the excitation potentials and pathways of the conduction system of the heart, the results often relating to anatomical disorders. For example, the presence of left ventricular hypertrophy is diagnosed if widened QRS complexes with large R waves in leads V5 and V6 with T wave inversion, and left axis deviation, is present. Such a condition may be due to overload of the chamber as seen in aortic stenosis or systemic hypertension. One might also expect atrial fibrillation to be the result of chronic left atrial hypertrophy that may have been caused by a stenosis of the mitral orifice.

The 12 lead diagnostic electrocardiogram is usually recorded within the frequency range of 0 or 0.05 to 100 Hz, and although it is considered adequate for routine evaluation the ECG does contain frequencies well above 800 Hz. The interpretation of these high frequency components has aroused much interest since the early 70s, when the recording technology became available, and whilst the non-invasive recording of the high frequency His bundle electrogram was pursued with much enthusiasm by many workers, the technique was not reliable and was therefore not clinical accepted.[24,25,26,27,28] This was mainly due to the limitations in the signal-to-noise ratio of amplification technology at that time. With advanced technology the reliability and accuracy has become much higher.

Whilst high frequency components contained in the initial portion of the QRS complex have been shown in acute myocardial infarction,[29] one of the areas in which analysis has proven useful has been in the measurement of *late potentials*. These high frequency, low amplitude, *(HFLA)* signals are found within or near the terminal portion of the QRS complex and are identified with those patients who are prone to inducement of spontaneous sustained re-entrant tachyarrhythmias, fibrillation and sudden death.

Sometimes known a *delayed depolarization potentials,* they are believed to represent late regional conduction within the borders of infarcted or aneurysmal myocardial tissue. Augmented with such diagnostic procedures as Holter recording, and radio-nuclide ejection fraction measurement they provide a reliable indication of risk.[30]

Acquisition and recording technique

Late potentials are extremely small electrograms of amplitude within the range of 1–10 μV, and are considerably lower in amplitude than the unseen artefact that is often present when recording the diagnostic electrocardiogram. Even barely visible alternating interference that is induced from power sources represents an amplitude of 5–10 μV.

FIGURE 54

The comparison of voltage ampltudes of various electrical signals as shown against a logarithmic scale.

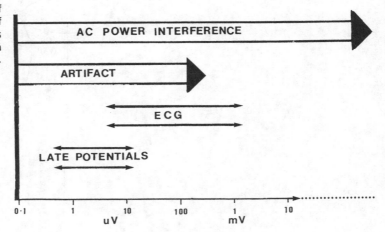

In order to analyse and record late potentials certain requirements must be met:

Firstly, the original ECG signals acquired from the body surface (usually *Frank orthogonal leads XYZ*) must be pure, of extremely high quality, free of muscle tremor, power noise, movement artefact or background noise of any kind.

Secondly, these ECG signals must be high-pass filtered to reduce the DC offset and further filtered to permit the analysis of the *HFLA* signals.

The method most favoured to carry out this task is *signal averaging*, a technique that will better the *signal/noise ratio* by decreasing the noise that is present within the baseline. This technique

FIGURE 55

The X (horizontal), Y (vertical) and Z (sagittal) leads of Frank

(Reproduced with kind permission of Marquette Electronics Inc.)

FRANK LEAD SET

ACQUISITION MODULE	FRANK LEADS	LOCATION
A1	H	SIDE OR BACK OF NECK
A2	E	*STERNUM MIDLINE
A3	I	*RIGHT MID AXILLARY LINE
A4	M	*CENTER THORACIC SPINE
V4	C	*MIDWAY BETWEEN ELECTRODES A AND E
V6	A	*LEFT MID AXILLARY LINE
LL	F	LEFT LEG

*These leads are in a horizontal plane at the level of the fifth intercostal space.

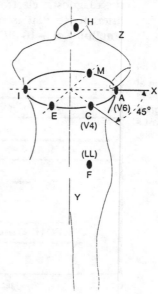

requires a series of ECG beats to be aligned and superimposed in order to reduce the baseline noise, from which an average waveform is generated.[31] Random noise is reduced by the square root of the number of beats averaged. Therefore the greater the number of beats analysed the better the signal to noise ratio. The averaged signals are aligned to allow the third condition to be met.

High gain amplification and analysis of the frequency components must be obtained. This technique known as *Fourier Filter Transform, or FFT* analyses the amplitudes of a series of sinusoidal waves that are contained within the ECG signal, which when added together reproduce the original signal. Once acquired, the final waveform is filtered and reconstructed to produce a visible electrogram of high gain that will indicate the presence or absence of late potentials.

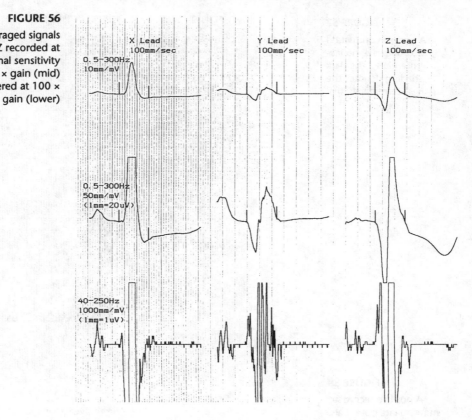

FIGURE 56

The averaged signals X,Y and Z recorded at normal sensitivity (upper), 5 × gain (mid) and filtered at 100 × gain (lower)

When assessing the presence of late potentials the following should be considered:

❑ Is the mean amplitude of the terminal 40 ms of the QRS vector less than 25 μV?

❑ Is the duration of the low amplitude signals, that is those less than 40 μV, greater than 40 ms?

FIGURE 57

A normal conduction recording. i.e. no late potentials . The dark shading denotes the terminal 40 ms.

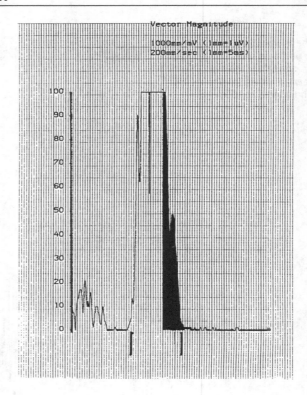

FIGURE 58

A positive recording showing late potentials.

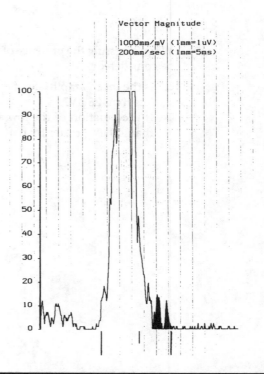

Further reading
❏ El-Sherif N, Gomes JAC, Restivo M, Mehra R. Late potentials and arrhythmogenesis. *Pace* 8: 440, 1985.

❏ Haberl R, Jilge G, Pulter R, Steinbeck G. Comparison of frequency and time domain analysis of the signal averaged electrocardiogram in patients with VT and CAD: methodologic evaluation and clinical revelance. *J Am Coll Cardiol* 12: 150, 1988.

3   *The Cath Lab*

Catheterisation of the heart is safe in experienced hands and today many centres are performing the technique according to guidelines recommended by the American College of Physicians and the American Hospital Association, as an *ambulatory* or out-patient procedure without the patient requiring overnight stay.[32]

The procedure is a very useful and important part of cardiac and circulatory diagnosis and, during the past decade, treatment. It involves the routine introduction of catheters and probes into the cardiovascular system via an artery or vein. Many of the types of catheters are known by their distinct distal shapes or those who developed them, e.g. "Pigtails", "Judkins", "Amplatz", "Double loop", "Curve right" "Curve left" "Cournand", "Sones", and are referred to as *guiding catheters* whilst others may have a single 45 ° distal curve with or without side holes.

The technologist plays a very important part as member of the cath team and is usually responsible for the recording of all haemodynamic monitoring. He or she must therefore have a good knowledge of the pathology of all the diseases that are likely to be investigated, know what is expected and be able to advise the physician of any unusual findings. Added to this he must be aware of the technical limitations of the equipment and be conversant with his or her role in the event of any emergency situations that may arise.

Catheterisation has many uses, and each may be grouped into either:

❑ *Diagnostic* i.e. to measure or analyse:
  • Pressures within the heart chambers, major vessels and pulmonary vasculature (by means of pressure transducers),
  • Blood oxygen saturations (using a density analyser),
  • Blood velocity and flow (catheter tipped transducers),
  • Cardiac output (thermodilution techniques),
  • Biopsy tissue from a transplanted or myopathic heart to detect early rejection or pathological changes (biopsy forceps).
  • The anatomy or function of heart chambers, coronary arteries or the left ventricle (by angiography),
  • The conduction system of the heart (electrophysiology studies); or

❑ *Therapeutic*, i.e. to:

- Dilate stenoses of the coronary vasculature (percutaneous transluminal coronary angioplasty (PTCA),
- Dilate stenotic valves (valvuloplasty),
- Infuse drugs (streptokinase, etc),
- Temporarily or permanently pace the heart (introduce electrode/s),
- Ablate the AV node (cryo probe, DC shock, RF current, etc),
- Counter pulsate (introduce an intra-aortic balloon),
- Remove foreign bodies,
- Open the atrial septum (Rashkind balloon septostomy),
- Close the atrial septum (patching techniques).

THE *X*-RAY IMAGER

To perform any of these diagnostic and therapeutic procedures it is necessary that an *x*-ray imaging device be used that will assist the physician in the routing and accurate positioning of the various catheters, electrodes and biopsy probes. To carry out this task certain pieces of equipment are necessary:

1. An *x*-ray translucent Table on which the patient is to lie.
2. An *x*-ray tube to generate the *x*-rays.
3. An image intensifier to transpose the x-radiation into an electron beam that may be minified (as opposed to magnified) and thereby increased in intensity.
4. An image distributor that will allow the image from the intensifier to be split or distributed through various ports to which a television camera or a high speed 35 mm film camera or both may be attached.
5. A transformer to supply the required voltages and currents.
6. A control desk at which energy settings may be made and controlled.

The *x*-ray imaging equipment may be single plane "C arm" unit, or duplicated to form the more commonly used bi-plane system: each allowing angiography to be performed in several planes, viz. anterior/posterior, lateral, caudal, etc.

Production of *x*-rays This is the function of the *x*-ray tube which basically consists of a wire filament, commonly known as the "heater"; a *cathode*, located around the heater; and an *anode,* all contained within a glass vacuumised tube or envelope. When an electric current is applied to the heater filament, electrons are released from the surface of the hot wire and contained within the boundaries of the cathode.

The application of a high voltage (up to 125 kV) between the cathode and the anode causes the electrons to accelerate towards the anode at a very high velocity that is dependent upon the voltage differential. The area of the anode (usually made of tungsten alloy) where the bombardment takes place, known as the *target,* is tangential to the direction of the electron beam. Whilst the vast majority of electrons are absorbed within the anode, generating heat, some of the electrons are deflected from the anode and converted into x-rays.

It is because of the enormous amount of heat generated during the anode bombardment, that a *rotating anode* tube is used. Rotating the anode at revolutions as high as 10 000 r/min, the heat is effectively dissipated over a much larger area. This allows the anode to operate at very high power ratings and longer exposure times that are often required during cardiac angiography, e.g. 125 kV at 500 mA.

The angle or tangent of the anode where the electron beam is focussed will influence the definition, or clarity, of the image. The smaller the spot where the beam is focussed, i.e. the focal spot of the tube, the better the image quality and the less the parallax. The nominal focal spot size is 0.6 and 1.0 mm, although it is often necessary to use smaller sizes for paediatric uses (0.3 and 0.8 mm). Tubes that allow double or triple focal spot sizes are commonly used in the catheterisation laboratory, having two or three circumferential tangents of the anode from which the x-rays are deflected. Typical triple tube nominal spot sizes are 0.3, 0.6, and 1.0mm.

For safety reasons the x-ray tube is normally mounted within a lead shield that has a window through which the x-rays pass. The lead shield containing the tube is immersed within a sealed container that is filled with oil. Heat generated by the tube causes convection currents within the oil which assists in its cooling. Located above and attached to the x-ray tube housing are *beam collimators* that eliminate the peripheral and more divergent portion of the x-ray beam by means of cones or diaphragms interposed in the path of the beam.

REMEMBER

❑ It is the voltage that determines the degree of penetration of the x-rays. The larger the patient the greater kV required.

❑ The current determines the electron flow within the tube and influences the image quality. The higher the current the better the definition.

❑ The focal spot size will, within limits, determine the sharpness of the image. The smaller spot size (fine focus) will produce a sharp image at the expense of a limited tube exposure, whereas the larger spot size (broad focus) will allow a large exposure to be used at the expense of the lack of geometric focusing. Much depends, however, on the exposure time e.g. a broad focus spot size will allow a sharp image when the time exposure is short enough to avoid subject movement. In other words, the geometric distortion may be generally poor but the motional sharpness good.

❑ An *x*-ray tube can only generate *x*-rays for a given time duration. Long periods of exposure will cause damage and/or a shortening of tube life, due to overheating.

The image intensifier

The next part of the *x*-ray chain is the image intensifier. Its job is to intensify the image from the *x*-ray tube by a system of optical convergence. The *x*-rays that have been directed towards the patient, who is lying on a table positioned between the *x*-ray tube and the image intensifier, are generated from a single radiating source. Once passed through the patient some of the radiation is inevitably scattered in all directions, which may harm nearby operators. One method of reducing the *scattered radiation* is to introduce a grid below the image intensifier. This is an arrangement of thin lead strips separated by a radiolucent material contained within a metal frame. Grids may be crossed, focussed, parallel, etc depending upon the configuration of the strips.

The image intensifier, or "I.I" as it is commonly known, consists of a large glass envelope in which is contained:

1. an *input phosphor* situated at the bottom end of the tube,
2. an *electron lens*, which is a series of electrically charged metal electrodes that surround the pattern of convergence, and
3. an *output phosphor* located at the top portion of the tube.

The input window of the intensifier tube is a highly transparent aluminium plate through which the *x*-rays pass before they reach the input phosphor. This convex phosphorescent screen (cesium iodide) absorbs the *x*-rays directed upon it, causing the emission of ultraviolet and visible radiation proportional to the intensity of the x radiation it receives.

On the concave side of the input phosphor a photo-electric metallic coating is painted that emits electrons proportional to the visible and ultraviolet radiation it receives. Known as the photocathode the coating is negatively charged.

The output phosphor is similar to the input phosphor except that it is smaller in diameter. It is a coating of a substance (commonly zinc cadmium) that will fluoresce when radiated with an electron beam, in a similar way that the screen of the cathode ray tube is made to fluoresce.

In order that the electrons emitted from the input phosphor are accelerated towards the output phosphor, a very high voltage differential of some 25 kV exists between them i.e. the photocathode (negative) and a conductive collar located around the output phosphor (positive), known as the photoanode. Complex electron optics, consisting of electrodes located between the photocathode and the photoanode and charged at a lower potential, control the divergence of the electron beam and also allow two or three image fields to be selected. Focusing is controlled by two cylindrical anodes that surround the electron beam.

The resultant image is of high resolution over the entire image area, free of astigmatism and possessing an extremely high intensity amplification in the range of 10 000–60 000.

FIGURE 59

Typical x-ray chain cnsisting a video and movie camera, video monitor, image distributor and x-ray tube.

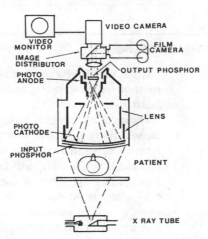

The image distributor This assembly is a light tight box, normally mounted above the output phosphor of the image intensifier. The image passes through a collimator lens (set at infinite focal length) into the distributor where it is split into three sources by means of mirrors. Each image source is transmitted through three separate ports located above and at the sides of the distributor box.

Approximately 20 % of the image intensity is distributed to a closed circuit television camera (CCTV) that is usually mounted above the distributor; and 80 % to a 35 mm high speed cine or a 100 mm spot film camera. The choice of cameras used may depend on personal preferences and/or clinical requirements. One or more video monitors may be serially connected to the TV camera.

X-rays generated during a catheterisation procedure are potentially harmful, especially to those operators who permanently employed in a catheterisation laboratory and who work in close proximity to the patient during the investigation.

1. Lead aprons should be worn by all within the room and thyroid shields and radiation opaque glasses worn by those near to the x-ray equipment.

2. All staff should be monitored for x radiation and wear a film badge at all times.

3. Unless necessary, do not stand close to the x-ray table.

REMEMBER

> Radiation decreases as the reciprocal square of the distance. Let us assume that one has unit radiation at unit distance. Now move 4 units away. The actual radiation level would be $\left(\frac{1}{4}\right)^2$ (the reciprocal square of the distance), or $\frac{1}{16}$ of the level of radiation at unit distance.

CATHETERISATION TECHNIQUES

Cardiac catheterisation is a general term that is used to describe the method of diagnosing and/or treating acquired and congenital heart diseases with the use of angiography and haemodynamic measuring equipment. Today, catheterisation of the heart encompasses many offshoot techniques that have developed in more recent years, all requiring the introduction of hollow catheters, electrical conductive insulated wires, balloons, etc. Although echocardiography has replaced much of the need for catheterisation, there is no doubt that the technique will be used for many years to come, especially for the diagnoses of some of the more complicated congenital diseases, for assessment of those patients requiring surgery, for evaluation of the conduction system, and more recently, to correct coronary artery and valvular obstruction.

Catheterisation of the right heart is usually performed via the femoral vein, and is indicated in the assessment of the following:

❑ intra-atrial or intra-ventricular left to right shunts or a combination of both,

❑ Diseases of the tricuspid valve.

❑ Diseases that involve the outflow tract of the right ventricle.

❑ Lesions of the pulmonary vascularture including hypertension, abnormal shunts either left to right or right to left.

❑ Restrictive or constrictive abnormalities involving the right ventricle.

❑ Left atrial pressure measurement through a puncture of the atrial septum.

❑ Endocardial biopsy for (i) the measurement of the degree of rejection after heart transplantation or (ii) to diagnose cardiomyopathy.

Most of the indications above would include a multitude of congenital as well as acquired lesions.

Catheterisation of the left heart is usually performed via one of the femoral arteries and is indicated in:

❑ Diseases involving the mitral and aortic valves.

❑ Unknown cause of LV failure.

❑ Restrictive or constrictive diseases of the left heart.

❑ Coarctation of the aorta.

❑ Obstructive diseases of the coronary arteries.

❑ Dissection of the aorta, etc.

Technique The catheters may be introduced by isolating the vessel after a cutdown (Sones method) or via a percutaneous approach. The most accepted technique is the percutaneous method of Seldinger. It is simple, quickly performed with local anaesthesia and without appreciable risk.

1. It requires a needle to be inserted into the vessel (Potts-Cournand).
2. Through the needle a short guide wire is introduced.
3. The needle is removed and a sheath set (dilator with sheath) fed over the guide wire into the vessel.
4. The sheath is advanced to its hub and the wire and dilator removed.
5. A syringe is attached to the hub of the sheath until the required catheter is introduced.

Percutaneous entry may be made via the subclavian, external jugular, femoral vein or via the femoral artery. A cutdown and exposure of the brachial vein is rarely performed.

Once inserted into the vessel, the catheter is gently pushed under x-ray guidance into the heart chambers, great vessels or the periphery of the lung fields. Several procedures may then be undertaken.

1. Pressures may be measured, by means of a transducer. (flow, velocity, valve gradients, shunts, anatomical disorders)
2. x-ray opaque dye may be infused under pressure. (shunts, abnormal anatomy, constrictions, incompetent valves, diseased vessels)
3. Samples of blood may be withdrawn and analysed.(shunts, haemoglobin, oxygen saturation)

4. A cold injectate may be infused. (cardiac output measurement)

5. A radioactive isotope may be infused. (shunts, abnormal pathways).

Let us now study some examples of the above common procedures.

Pressures The measurement of pressures within the chambers and great vessels is the most reliable single method of assessment of severity of anatomical or vascular disorders. This is especially so in the congenital heart disease group of patients when complicated lesions are to be diagnosed.

Example: one of the most common congenital lesions is *tetralogy of Fallot (1888)*, accounting for 66 % of all congenital heart defects accompanied with clubbing of the finger nails, polycythemia and central cyanosis, This "blue baby" disease has four main disorders:

1. Pulmonary stenosis
2. Ventricular septal defect
3. Overriding of the aorta
4. Right ventricular enlargement

There are many grades of the disease. 50 % have stenosis of the infundibular tract, 33 % of the pulmonary valve and the remainder both infundibular and pulmonary stenoses.

A VSD is present in varying degrees and permits desaturated blood from the right ventricle to escape across the septum to the left ventricle so causing central cyanosis. The other contributing factor to the cyanosis is the "override" of the aorta, which is actually dextroposed, for its root is displaced to the right side thereby permitting right ventricular blood to readily enter it. The right ventricle is enlarged due to pressure overload in having to pump against the normal systemic pressure contained within the left ventricle and aorta.

At cardiac catheterisation, blood pressures within the two ventricles are always found to be identical, and when the pulmonary artery is entered, an extremely high pressure gradient exists across the pulmonary valve. Aortic pressure can often be measured as the catheter passes through the septum or into the override. Fortunately, open heart surgery is able to offer much relief for most patients with this disease, for both the override of the aorta and the VSD can be corrected and the stenosed infundibulum resected and/or the stenotic valve relieved.

Pressure measurements taken from each chamber supply information of the severity of the physiological disorder and to a lesser extent the abnormal anatomy.

Normal heart pressures in mm Hg

Site	Range sys/dia	Mean	% O₂ sat
IVC	4/1	1–7	80
SVC	4/1	1–7	70
RA	7/1	4	75
RV	28/0	—	75
MPA	28/5	8–22	75
PCW	—	4–12	96–100
LA	10/2	4–12	96
LV	150/2	-	96
AO	150/60	70–100	96

In the adult, O_2 saturations within the IVC are invariably higher than in the SVC, due to extra demand of oxygen to the brain, although the reverse situation is commonly seen in the infant

FIGURE 60

The normal waveforms and pressures of the heart chambers

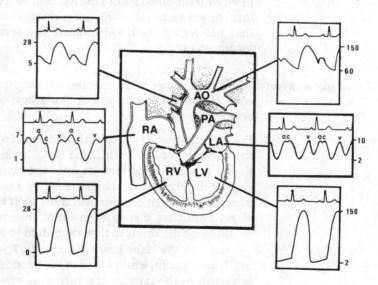

Angiography Angiography involves the infusion of an *x*-ray opaque substance via a catheter into the chambers of the heart, the coronary arteries (coronary angiography) or great vessels. Modern methods of imaging allow the substance to be clearly seen on a video monitor screen as it is transported through the heart.

Permanent storage of the image may be recorded on video tape or on a digital storage system. A 35 mm film of the angiogram that is recorded on a high speed movie camera attached to the image distributor of the x-ray column, is often recorded for long term storage, comprehensive study and later audience viewing.

Angiography is of special importance when viewing stenotic vessels, detecting shunts within the heart and across adjacent vessels and for the assessment of valvular stenosis or incompetence.

Example

Imagine a patient with incompetence of the aortic valve who has a catheter that has been introduced into the femoral artery, the tip of which is located within the ascending aorta distal to the aortic valve. A high pressure injection of x-ray opaque dye, or as it is often called, "contrast medium", is given through the catheter and serial recordings taken as the dye occupies the root of the aorta (sinus of Valsalva).

During the diastolic phase, when the heart is relaxed and therefore has minimal restriction to blood flow, some dye will be seen to enter the two coronary arteries, also some of the dye that has diffused with the blood within the root will be seen to regurgitate back into the left ventricle — whence it came. The density of the media that has regurgitated will indicate the severity of the valvular incompetence.

Blood gas analyses

Blood gas analyses will assist the cardiologist in assessing the presence of abnormal pathways of blood flow within the heart and adjacent vessels.

Example: Imagine a patient with a VSD who is catheterised and has the catheter located within the distal pulmonary artery. Withdrawal of serial blood samples from the pulmonary artery and in each of the chambers back to the RA, and their subsequent measurement of oxygen content, will show a left to right blood flow, or *shunt*, (assuming there are no other anatomical anomalies that would cause the shunt to flow from right to left).

Blood in the right heart is normally 70–75 % saturated with oxy-haemoglobin, whilst blood in the left side is normally 95–98 % saturated. As the catheter is slowly withdrawn and blood samples taken from each chamber through the right heart, they would reveal a small, moderate, or large increase in saturation in the pulmonary artery and the right ventricle, indicating a flow of blood from the left ventricle. The amount of increase will directly depend on the amount of flow from left to right. Typical saturations might be 70 % in the right atrium and 80 % in the right ventricle and pulmonary artery.

In the cath lab the samples are usually taken from following specific sites and subsequently analysed.

1. SVC
2. RA/SVC junction
3. Mid RA
4. Low RA
5. Low RV
6. Body RV
7. RV Outflow Tract
8. MPA
9. RPA
10. LPA, and
11. Wedged Pulmonary Capillary.

Cardiac output measurements See "Cardiac output measurements" on page 104.

The vast majority of patients seen in the adult cardiac catheterisation laboratory have ischemic heart disease and require coronary angiography to demonstrate the severity of the disease. In addition, selective angiography of the left ventricle may be required to evaluate its size, wall motion and thickness and also of the aorta if stenosis or incompetence is suspected.

PERCUTANEOUS TRANSLUMINAL CORONARY ANGIOPLASTY (PTCA)

PTCA[33] is routinely performed on patients with single or multi-vessel disease in many advanced cardiac centres of the world and has now become more competitive than ever to bypass surgery (CABG) as a means of revascularisation of stenotic coronary vessels. It is estimated that the success of the procedure is well over 90 %. The remaining 10 % is due to (a) failure to cross the lesion with either the guide wire or catheter, which accounts for some 50 % of cases; (b) sudden re-closure of the lesion, 45 %; or (c) failure to dilate the lesion, 3 %.

The technique of angioplasty is relatively simple, although there is no doubt that it requires considerable experience and skill to perform. It entails the defining of the coronary vessels by the injection of contrast media in order to determine the origin of the occluded vessel(s), the insertion of a coaxial guiding wire over which a catheter is introduced that has a small balloon situated at its distal tip. Once located within the stenotic coronary artery, inflation of the balloon causes the atheromatous substance to be compressed against the wall of the vessel which has the effect of increasing its lumen. With the aid of bi-plane angiography operating in specific radiological views, e.g. RAO, LAO, LAT, CR and CA, and with the use of the correct guiding wires to allow crucial placement of the balloon it is often possible to dilate small distal vessels.

Although the risks of the procedure are relatively low, the incidence of re-stenosis is unfortunately high, especially in those patients with multi-vessel disease (20–40 %).

PERCUTANEOUS BALLOON MITRAL VALVULOPLASTY (PBMV)

A similar technique to PTCA, valvuloplasty entails the use of a catheter that has an hour-glass shaped balloon at its distal end which, when located through the stenotic valve, is inflated causing the commissures to open. The technique has become popular as an alternative to closed heart mitral commissurotomy and in some instances, replacement of the aortic valve. It is commonly used in paediatric cardiology.

The technologist should realise that the technique of cardiac catheterisation may involve many different procedures. The number and the type depending upon the kind of lesion or lesions present. Much depends on the requirements of the investigating physician or surgeon, who must conclude a diagnosis and/or correct the abnormalities.

FIGURE 61

The pressure differences across the mitral valve before and after valvuloplasty. Normally the left atrial and left ventricular pressures during diastole are equal.

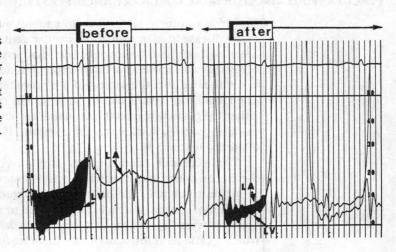

THE BLOOD PRESSURE TRANSDUCER

Long term continuous recording of blood pressure is measured by means of a transducer, a device that will transform or change one type of energy into another. The energy may be electrical, pneumatic, hydraulic, mechanical, light, ultrasound or any other physical phenomenon. Most transducers convert a physical entity into electrical signals that can be measured by a suitable recording device.

The pressure-sensing transducer commonly found in the hospital environment utilizes a membrane or diaphragm that is displaced when pressure is applied upon it. It is therefore displacement and not pressure that is actually measured. The transducer membrane may be considered as a spring-mass system having a single degree of freedom as shown in figure 62. It is a mass suspended by a spring. Any downward movement of mass M will cause it to be returned by the spring. Connected to the mass are two helical dashpots which restrain periodic oscillations of the spring-mass system.

FIGURE 62
Analogy of pressure transduction (see text)

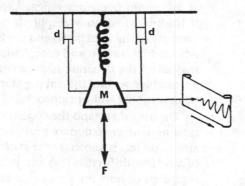

The behaviour of the fluid-filled membrane transducer may also be considered as a system that is constrained to a single degree of freedom with mass, compliance and damping.

Mass of a transducer system usually refers to the mass of fluid contained within the pressure dome, connecting tubing and catheters etc., plus the effective mass which includes the moving mass of the membrane proper.

Compliance refers to the elastic properties of the membrane, and to a smaller degree those of the catheter and/or connective tubing. *Damping* is the means of dissipating the energy of an oscillatory system to reduce its amplitude. It usually refers to the viscosity of the fluid-filed system. Damping in a water filled system may, therefore be increased by:

❑ An increase in the viscosity of the fluid link between pressure source and transducer, e.g. blood;

❑ Increase in the friction of the system, e.g. a constriction in the bore of the connective tubing, narrow bore needles, or

❑ By an increase in compliance, e.g. the presence of air bubbles within the fluid system or by the introduction of a small opening through which fluid may escape.

The ideal requirements of a transducer may be summarised as follows:

1. Adequate frequency response
2. Sensitivity
3. Stability
4. Simplicity

It is obvious that any system that measures a variable function must be able to respond adequately to the highest frequency component of that function. The fidelity to which the system will respond is known as its *dynamic response*. It is the ratio of amplitude to pressure at maximum frequency range. Adequate dynamic response refers to the linear frequency/amplitude ratio, (effected by the inertia and viscosity of the fluid mass) and the linear frequency/phase lag ratio (effected by friction and compliance of the system). Many factors may affect the dynamic response of a pressure system, e.g., micro air bubbles within the tubing, long tubing lengths, high compliance tubing and/or stopcocks.

On the other hand the system must also be able to respond to slow moving or stationary pressures and the fidelity to which it is able to do this is known as the *static response*, and refers to freedom of base-line drift (stability) and its response to any static pressure regardless of how the pressure is applied (uniqueness). Therefore, the transducer, associated amplifier to which it is connected and the recording galvanometer must each faithfully reproduce the amplitude and contour of the applied pressure pulse. In order to achieve this end the transducer diaphragm must be easily deformed or lax so that it may respond to slow moving vibrations. Conversely the membrane must be taut and rigid so that it may respond to rapid and very small amplitude vibrations. These two properties are directly opposed and therefore in the construction of a transducer there has to be much compromise.

The ability of a transducer to accurately respond to rapidly applied serial pressures is a function of its natural frequency and is said to possess a *high natural frequency*. On the other hand a transducer having a very lax membrane will not be able to respond to rapid pressure changes and will therefore have a *low natural frequency*.

The damped natural frequency of a particular transducer membrane can be mathematically calculated from the formula:

$$fo = \frac{1}{2\pi}\sqrt{\frac{E\pi r^2}{Ln}}$$

where:

fo is the natural frequency (Hz)

E is the modulus of elasticity of the membrane (dynes × cm^5)

r is the radius of the system (cm)

L is the length of the system (cm)

n is the viscosity of the fluid (poise units)

From this equation it can be clearly seen that to achieve a high natural frequency it is necessary that the radius be large and the length and viscosity small. Much will depend on the modulus of elasticity which is determined by the properties of the membrane material. It may be defined as the unit force required to produce a unit volume displacement in the transducer.

In order to further understand what is meant by the term "natural frequency" it is necessary to consider the requirements of the transducer membrane in relation to the pressures it must measure.

The pressure changes that occur within the vascular system may extend to the limits of approximately –5 to 300 mm Hg and the frequency range of these pressure contours may exceed 40 Hz, depending on heart rate. Analyses has shown that the cardiovascular pressure pulse is composed of a series of simple sine waves with a frequency of up to the 10th harmonic of the fundamental and that accurate registration of pressure pulses can be accomplished by any system having a satisfactory uniform dynamic response that is related to heart rate.

This all means that at a heart rate of 120 beats per minute i.e. 2 per second (the fundamental frequency), the highest frequency contained within the pressure contour would be 20 Hz which is the 10th harmonic of the fundamental frequency. (For ordinary clinical purposes a frequency response flat to 20 Hz is adequate. However, in specialised laboratories when measurements such as dP/dt or arterial impedance is required to be measured by Fourier analyses a higher response e.g. flat to 100 Hz, may be required).

There are of course other factors that will affect the response characteristics of the complete pressure system:

❑ *External tubing.* Frequency response of the pressure system will be lowered if the externally applied tubing is too long, too small internal diameter or made of material that is too elastic.

- ❑ *Viscosity of fluid* within the system. Frequency response will be lowered if the viscosity is increased (e.g. blood) or if minute air bubbles are present.
- ❑ The *use of stopcocks* will decrease the frequency response of the system due to internal diameter mismatching.
- ❑ *Coiling of catheter tubing* lines should be avoided to prevent minor lowering of frequency response.
- ❑ *Recording apparatus.* This essentially relates to the frequency response of the galvanometer which must be able to linearly respond well above the frequencies of the applied transducer pressures.

Certain distortions are often recorded from within the cardiovascular system of comparatively high frequencies. These are caused by the free undamped vibrations occurring within the catheter and are maintained by intrinsic influences to which the catheter is exposed during the catheterisation procedure. Commonly known as *catheter whip* it is often seen when the catheter crosses, or is near to, the pulmonary valve.

Damping of these artefactual oscillations may be achieved electrically, by imposing a capacitance network in the system; or hydraulically, by imposing a resistance to fluid flow between the catheter and the transducer.

Most pressure amplifiers have a variable damping range switch incorporated enabling the operator to dampen artefacts without affecting either the amplitude or delay of the pressure. By electrically overdamping, mean pressures may also be recorded this way. Damping may also be imposed hydraulically by the use of various size constrictions introduced between the catheter and the transducer or by the use of a simple needle valve.

One manufacturer (Spectromed, USA) has developed a fixed damping device that may be inserted in-line with the catheter. It consists of a plastic chamber in which a pliable silicone diaphragm is housed and is very useful in general situations i.e. critical care, cath lab, where an increased compliance is required to eliminate systolic overshoot or to reduce catheter whip. Being a fixed damping device, the technologist should be aware of its limitations, especially when used in conjunction with other means of damping. It should be used with caution whenever lag and amplitude are of critical importance, unless these parameters have been previously measured.

In order to accurately record physiological pressures the transducer and associated equipment must respond with equal amplitude throughout the entire range of frequencies that the pressure contour co..t.ains, provided that a constant amplitude input pressure is applied to the transducer membrane. Therefore the amplitude or sensitivity of the system must be equal within the range (or bandwidth) of zero to the maximal frequency component of the pressure contour. Conversely, the frequency components of the pressure pulse should be within the frequency bandwidth of the catheter-manometer system.

For example, a sinusoidal pressure variation of x units amplitude will, when applied to a transducer system, respond with a constant amplitude of x units irrespective of frequency up to the ideal maximum physiological component. For most manometric investigations 25 Hz at a damping factor of 0.6 is usually satisfactory.

> However, it is unfortunate that the catheter/manometer system acts as a low pass filter that tends to attenuate high frequency components.

The required range of response of the transducer is dependent upon the heart rate of the patient i.e. the fundamental frequency, and the type of pulse contour it records. It is not difficult to imagine that a hyperkinetic aortic pulse would contain higher frequency components than the normal aortic contour. The rapid upstroke of the aortic pulse might well require a range beyond the 30th harmonic of its fundamental frequency.

FIGURE 63

The response curves of a membrane oscillatory system that is subject to various degrees of damping.
(*fo* is the natural frequency of the membrane)

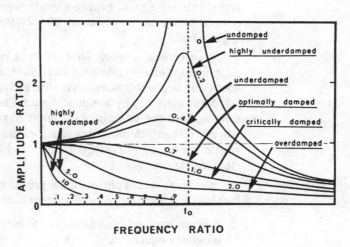

The *undamped natural frequency* is the resonant frequency at which the system will oscillate with no damping imposed upon it (i.e frictionless). It varies as the square root of the ratio of pressure to volume and is termed the *volume elastic coefficient*. As damping is increasingly imposed the amplitude ratio decreases throughout its damped natural frequency range until a point of *optimal damping*

is attained. Such a degree of damping forces the system to attenuate 22 % of its natural frequency and at a condition when the frequency/amplitude response is "flat". Optimal damping therefore affords the most constant relationship of amplitude throughout the widest frequency range. It is also 70 % of the damping imposed on the system at its *critically damped* level. Critical damping forces a system to attenuate some 50 % at its natural frequency, being the amount of damping that will just prevent critical limitation of its amplitude. Further increase in damping will result in a highly damped system that will attenuate rapidly with little or no dynamic response.

It can be seen that a system having a natural frequency of 200 Hz will have a linear amplitude ratio/frequency response up to 60 Hz at a level of critical damping. 60 Hz being a point at which the response curve begins to fall. In this example at 0.3 of its natural frequency.

At the other extreme a system having a natural frequency of only 30 Hz would at a level of *critical damping* only respond flat up to 9 Hz.

It has been shown that in order to record pressure contours of the vascular system without distortion, it is necessary that all frequency components are delayed equally so that they maintain the same relationship to one another. It is a physical misfortune that any oscillatory system having a single degree of freedom will produce a phase lag response of 90° as the natural frequency is approached.

At an *optimal damping level* (70 % of critical) there is a linear relationship between phase lag and frequency. Distortion will occur above and below this linear level with increase or decrease in phase lag. Most users of physiological pressure recording apparatus will have noticed the amount of lag imposed on a pressure waveform when it is highly damped due to either the presence of air bubbles within the system (increase compliance), blood, or by hydraulic or electrical damping.

In order to record physiological pressures accurately, it is important that a transducer recorder system has:

1. A linear frequency/amplitude ratio beyond the range of physiological frequencies,
2. A linear frequency/phase lag response which is only obtained at an optimal level of damping,
3. Sensitivity — a quality of linear response to a stepwise increase of static pressure and to a slow pressure function,
4. Stability — meaning freedom from base-line and calibration factor drift.

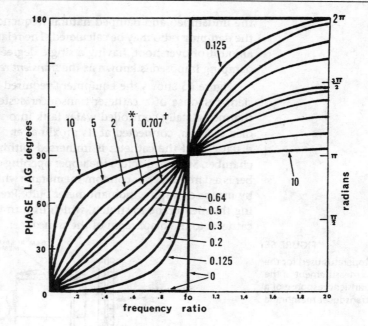

FIGURE 64

The relationship between the phase lag and frequency of an oscillating membrane system.

* the point of critical damping

\+ the point of optimal damping

fo the undamped natural frequency

Unfortunately few physiological laboratories are in possession of equipment that can accurately assess all these aforementioned parameters. As no transducer can be expected to retain these requirements throughout its life, periodic checkout is essential.

However, it is possible for the technologist to determine the condition of the complete recording system within the accuracy demanded or, within certain limitations, without the use of test equipment.

By the application of an instantaneous pressure wave to the transducer membrane and recording of the resultant waveform it is possible to roughly check the response of the system. A simple method is by the rapid turning of a two-way stopcock connected to the transducer, between atmospheric zero and a pressure of 100 mm Hg. The resultant waveform will reveal an undamped, critically or overdamped system. The undamped trace will show a large overshoot that will; return rapidly to its actual pressure level. The critically damped trace will show a fractional or nil overshoot i.e. the galvanometer will respond readily and instantly to its applied pressure by an absolute "squarewave".

In the overdamped recording a rounded waveform is seen indicating that time is required for the system to respond to such a sudden pressure wave.[34]

This method does not, however, give an indication of the frequency/ amplitude ratio nor an accurate assessment of the degree of damping of the system. However, from the resultant curves both the undamped and damped natural frequency of the system and the damping ratio may be calculated. The relationship between the amount of overshoot, having a single degree of freedom, and the damping imposed is known as the *transient response*.

Figure 65 shows the equipment required to measure the transient response of a catheter-transducer system.[35] It consists of a thermostatically controlled water tank into which is coiled a cardiac catheter, connected at its proximal end to a transducer. The distal end of the catheter is immersed within a partly filled fluid chamber. Stretched across the upper opening of the pressure chamber is a dam rubber or condom membrane which may be distended by means of a sphygmomanometer bulb. Pressure is applied causing the membrane to stretch, which in turn is transmitted via the catheter to the diaphragm of the transducer.

FIGURE 65

Apparatus used for the measurement of the transient response of a transducer membrane

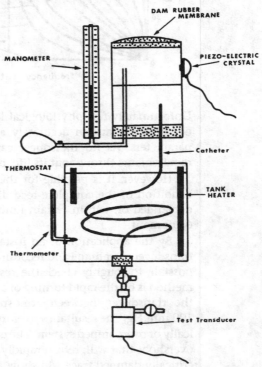

Puncture of the taught rubber membrane produces a sudden release of pressure within the chamber and corresponding fall on the transducer membrane. The implosion is recorded by the piezo-electric crystal that indicates instantaneous release of the chamber pressure. The recorded waveform will produce a "square wave" contour which may be analysed.

Figure 66 shows the pattern produced by an underdamped system having a 25 % overshoot and a damped natural frequency of

FIGURE 66
Transient response
showing how the
resultant curve is
analysed for overshoot
and natural frequency.

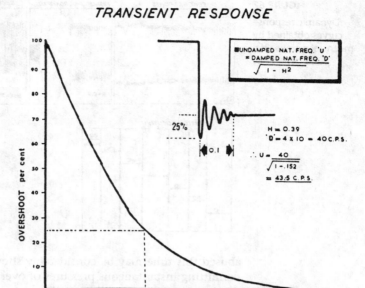

TRANSIENT RESPONSE

40 Hz. From the formula and graph both the degree of damping and the undamped natural frequency can be calculated. The use of the piezo-electric sound when simultaneously recorded with the sudden onset of pressure decrease will enable the operator to assess the transmission delay time of the system from catheter tip to transducer.

The most convenient method to measure the frequency/amplitude ratio and the frequency/phase lag response of the transducer recorder system is with the use of a sinusoidal hydraulic pulse generator. With this instrument a sine wave pressure may be applied directly to the transducer. By increasing the generated frequency from zero to a range beyond the natural frequency of the test transducer it is possible to accurately ascertain the linearity of the system. Figure 67 shows the effect of damping on a transducer when subject to oscillations that vary in frequency from such a hydraulic generator. Displayed on a cathode ray oscilloscope the phase lag and frequency response may easily be measured.

Sensitivity may be measured without the aid of elaborate equipment and is a comparatively simple procedure which should be carried out at frequent intervals throughout the life of the apparatus. It should be remembered that it is not uncommon for transducers to become statically alinear after prolonged use due to internal stresses and strains imposed on its diaphragm. If the transducer is

FIGURE 67

Dynamic response curves obtained by means of a sinusoidal pulse generator.

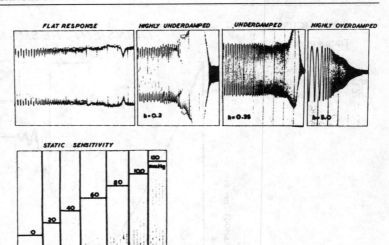

abused this time may be considerably shortened. The practice of permitting instantaneous pressures of over 300 mm Hg to hit the diaphragm when flushing the catheter should be avoided.

Static linearity problems may not be due to the transducer alone as such faults may occur within the amplifier or recorder. The purpose of a linearity check is to make sure that the deflection of the recording device moves in direct relationship to the applied pressure. For example if the sensitivity is so adjusted that a pressure of 100 mm Hg will deflect the recording mechanism 4 cm. then it would be natural to assume that a pressure of 25 mm Hg would deflect 1 cm, and a pressure of 75 mm Hg; 3 cm, etc. If this is so then the system is said to be linear. In checking it is necessary to first calibrate the system by applying pressure in steps of 10 mm Hg until 150 mm Hg is reached. This should be done on a suitable sensitivity range and each increment of pressure recorded in a stepwise fashion. Thus the final figure corresponding to 150 mm Hg would reach 6 cm from the base line (assuming our original calibration to be 100 mm Hg/4 cm). This procedure should be repeated on ALL ranges of sensitivity. On high ranges a saline column should be used.

It is also important that comparative tests of ranges of sensitivity be made, for although a system may be linear, its pressure/deflection sensitivity may alter on any range of amplification.

For example, a pressure of 50 mm Hg applied to the transducer set at a pressure range of 100 should deflect the recorder 2 cm. That same pressure should deflect the recorder 1 cm if the range is changed to 200. Similarly the deflection should be 4 cm if the range is 50 and 8 cm if the range is 25.

Stability refers to the static accuracy of the transducer in relation to its zero baseline drift. Drift of the transducer output with zero input should ideally be absent. However drift occurs in all transducer-manometer systems to a lesser or greater degree and is normally expressed in mm Hg per unit time. A zero drift of 10 mm Hg/min would be completely unsuitable for pressure measurement of the atrial contour and references to true zero would have to continually be made. On the other hand a drift of 10 mm Hg/hour would be negligible. Zero drift is often due to temperature change and is often referred to by some manufacturers as the *thermal coefficient* of the transducer.

Calibration factor drift refers to drift in the sensitivity and subsequent repeated calibrations should not detract from the original factors. If the static response of a positively applied pressure differs in output to the same negatively applied pressure, the transducer is said to exhibit hysteresis.

TYPES OF PRESSURE MEASURING DEVICES

Pressure transducers are generally classified according to the method of transference of the pressure pulse into a signal that is acceptable to a recording system. As the vast majority of recorders require an electrical signal in either analogue or digital form, it is necessary to change the pressure pulses received from the patient into some form of electrical signal.

The *capacitive* transducer[36] makes use of variations of the dielectric distance of a capacitor. When two metal plates are separated by an insulator, or dielectric, they constitute an electrical capacitor and when incorporated in an electrical circuit will maintain an electrical charge upon them. The ratio of the charge to the potential difference between the plates is termed "capacitance".

The charge of current on the plates may be varied by the :

☐ Area of the plates
☐ Distance between the plates and
☐ Material between the plates (the dielectric)

In the capacitive transducer use is made of the distance between the plates and as one of the plates forms part of the transducer membrane, pressure upon it causes the distance from it to the other plate to vary. As part of a radio-frequency alternating circuit, the capacitor is caused to behave somewhat similarly to the variable resistance of a DC circuit.

Although the system has a high natural frequency it is prone to temperature variations and inclined to be unstable. In all other respects however, it is an excellent robust transducer.

The *inductive* transducer utilises a magnetic iron core that is able to move within a wire coil thereby causing an electromagnetic force (EMF) to be induced within the coil. The iron core is attached to a pressure diaphragm which when displaced within the coil produces a variation of induced current proportional to the applied pressure.

This method of pressure transference has the advantage of a high natural frequency with good baseline stability and has for many years been used in catheter-tipped devices. The advantage of this application of the inductive transducer over external transducers is that motion artefact or "catheter whip" is avoided. The major disadvantage is that a zero reference pressure level cannot be assessed unless used in conjunction with a conventional external transducer system.

By far the most popular of all types is the *resistive* transducer or "strain gauge". Its operation is entirely due to the fact that when a wire is stretched its electrical resistance increases. Resistance is therefore affected by its length, cross sectional area and the material of which the wire is made. It may be classified into two distinct types, each employed for the transfer of strain (created by pressure) upon a material into electrical current: *bonded* and *unbonded*.

Bonded
In the bonded gauge[37] the resistance wire is firmly cemented or bonded to the material that is being measured for strain. The wire or wires may be cemented throughout the entire length of, for example, a steel girder, so that bending of the girder will cause the wire to stretch and its resistance to alter. A voltage applied between the two ends of the wire will produce a proportional change of electrical current. Force transducers, similarly constructed may be used to measure myocardial function when attached directly to the wall of the heart. The same principle is applied in the solid state silicon transducer, which is in essence, a resistive circuit that is cemented to an elastic material that is stressed by pressure.

Both stress (applied force/unit area) and strain (increase in length/ unit length) may be measured by means of the unbonded gauge although the basic construction is that of a strain element.

Unbonded
The unbonded gauge[38] has during the past years lost some of its popularity in the field of medicine. It differs from the bonded type in so far as it consists of two pairs of wires, coiled and assembled in such a manner that displacement of a membrane connected to them causes one pair to stretch and the other to relax. The two pairs of the wires are not bonded to the material under stress but are attached by retaining lugs. Because of the delicacy of the wire used it is possible to obtain large changes of current. The resistance wires form part of a *Wheatstone bridge* network.

The resistive transducer has the great advantage of possessing high stability and is therefore suitable for long-term continuous pressure recording. Base line drift is minimal and because of its construction it is relatively insensitive to temperature fluctuations. The only disadvantage is its low natural frequency. Nevertheless it is by far the most widely used transducer in cardiovascular medicine. Unbonded strain gauges located at the tip of a cardiac catheter offer freedom from motion artefact and lag of catheter response.

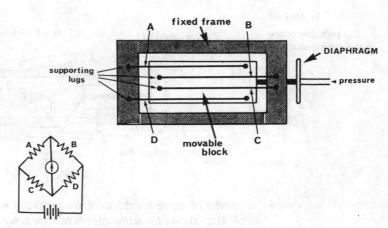

FIGURE 68

The unbonded strain gauge. The inset illustrates how the wires are connected that form the Wheatstone Bridge

Figure 68 illustrates the construction of the unbonded strain gauge transducer. Wires A, B, C and D represent the two pairs of strain wires connected at their one end to a movable block and at the other to a fixed frame. As pressure is applied to the diaphragm it causes the movable block to slide, so tightening wires B and C whilst relaxing wires A and D. The inset shows the electrical analogue of the transducer consisting of four resistance wires arranged in the form of a bridge. As wires B and C are stretched — causing the resistance to increase, and wires A and D are relaxed — causing the resistance to decrease, the bridge will become unbalanced and the current from the battery will cause the needle to deflect from its zero balanced condition proportional to (*a*) the change of resistance of the bridge and (*b*) the applied pressure to the diaphragm of the transducer. The complete arrangement is commonly known as a Wheatstone bridge network.

Solid-state transducers With the advances of silicon strain gauge technology since the early 1960s, solid state transducers, whether disposable or re-usable are today commonplace. They are, in effect, bonded transducers having their silicon and piezoresistor transducer elements etched into a silicon microchip by a photolithographic process — the equivalent of the four resistive wires of the unbonded strain gauge. Because the silicon chip on which the resistive elements are etched has good elastic properties and is very responsive to small pressure changes that are transmitted from the diaphragm, it has a high sensitivity and little or no hysteresis. These two qualities and the size of the diaphragm allow it to have a low displacement volume and a good frequency response.

FIGURE 69

The principle of the solid state transducer

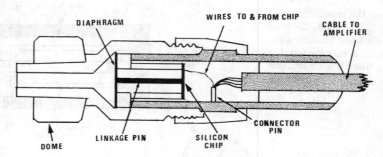

Some of these transducers are provided with a compensation cable that allows for adjustments of *impedance matching*. The transducer has a high impedance and if connected to a low impedance monitor could give erroneous recordings. Although most of the new generation monitors have high input impedances it is *important* to ensure that transducer and monitor are compatible.

Figure 69 illustrates how the pressure from the diaphragm is transmitted to the silicon chip causing it and the elements which are etched upon it to be stressed. As the pressure changes so does the resistance of the elements proportionally change, and as these form part of the Wheatstone bridge circuit, changes of electrical current will similarly take place. These changes of current are transmitted from the chip to connector pins via hair-like wires. A standard electrical cable is connected to the pins which conducts the varying electrical signals to a suitable amplifier and recorder.

It should be noted that whatever type of transducer is used, it has to be "excited" from a DC source (battery) or from an *AC carrier amplifier*. Both provide the energy necessary to operate the Wheatstone bridge. Most pressure amplifiers operate from AC power and produce a high frequency alternating signal in order to excite the Wheatstone bridge. (Remember, a high frequency signal of approximately 10 000 Hz, will behave like a DC source in a purely resistive circuit.)

The technologist who is considering the purchase of a transducer whether it be reusable or disposable, would be well advised to read the technical specifications that are available from the manufacturers. Although there are many similarities in the properties, he should be aware of some of the more important differences that various manufacturers offer.

- *Operating pressure range* in mm Hg. This refers to the limits of pressure over which the transducer will linearly cover. It is important that its range extends well beyond physiological pressures both in a negative and positive direction.

- *Sensitivity* in uV/V/mm Hg refers to the ability of the transducer to respond to the pressure it receives. Most transducers have a sensitivity in the order of 5uv/V/mm Hg.

- *Excitation voltage* in volts AC or DC is the potential required to excite the bridge. The figure specified (usually less than 12 volts DC) should not be exceeded and the transducer should be compatible with the corresponding amplifier with which it is to be used. If AC voltage is used the RMS value is usually 5 kHz.

- *Frequency response* measured in herz is the maximum flat frequency at which the transducer can operate. Many can fulfil responses of over 400 Hz.

- *Overpressure* in mm Hg is the maximum pressure which can be applied to the diaphragm without causing it to distort or be damaged in any way. It is well to remember that even the act of taking off or putting on a stopcock without previously opening the transducer diaphragm to atmosphere can create extremely high pressures that may subsequently damage the transducer. However, some transducers are able to withhold pressures of up to 6000 mm Hg or more.

- *Zero thermal coefficient* in mm Hg/°C relates to the thermal drift of the transducer i.e. the number of mm Hg the recording will drift per degree Celcius temperature rise or fall. This figure should be less than 0.5 mm Hg/°C.

- *Non-linearity* or *hysteresis error* is usually measured as a percentage of full scale deflection (FSD) and should be below 2 %.

- *Volume displacement* in mm^3/100 mm Hg is the amount of volume change within the dome when 100 mm Hg of pressure is applied. Usually less than 0.4 although many disposable units may be as low as 0.04 mm^3/100 mm Hg.

- *Defibrillation withstand* is the amount of DC shock that the transducer will accept without damage. It should be in excess of 6000 V or 5 repeated discharges within a period of 5 min.

- *Leakage current* should be well below 5uA at 115 V 60 Hz RMS and 10 μA at 220 V 50 Hz RMS.

Throw away or use again? The decision whether to use permanent or disposable transducers will depend on the type of usage, experience of the operators and in some instances, the costs.

Perhaps in the catheterisation laboratory where trained technologists are daily operating pressure equipment, it might be more economical and reliable to use permanent types. On the other hand in an intensive care unit where many changes of medical and nursing personnel take place, and where patients are sometimes moved to other areas, disposable units with transfer cables or modules should be considered.

Most permanent transducers can be used well over 500 times when handled carefully by experienced technical staff.

Before making a decision, ask yourself.

❑ Is the transducer protected from DC shock that exceeds the maximum output of commercial defibrillators?

❑ What is the leakage current (measured in uA at a specified voltage)?

❑ Has the transducer a zero offset? If so what is the value?

❑ Does the output impedance of the transducer match the amplifier?

❑ Is the interface cable fully shielded to minimise electrical interference?

❑ If cost is important, don't forget each transducer requires a transparent polycarbonate dome and may require a cable.

MEASUREMENT OF CARDIAC OUTPUT

It is well known that the heart has a relatively minimal effect on the normal regulation of cardiac output[39] and at rest it will discharge against a wide range of pressures, whatever venous blood is returned to it. The heart functions like a double pump, the volume of blood pumped per minute is the product of stroke volume and heart rate e.g. if the stroke volume is 60 ml and the heart rate 100 bpm, the cardiac output (CO) would be 6 litres/minute. It is because the peripheral vessels are small and offer considerable resistance to blood flow, that the heart has to generate a pressure of ±100 mm Hg to maintain circulation of blood through the arteries, arterioles, capillaries and back to the heart via the veins. The distribution of blood however, is controlled by each of the organs receiving it, each regulating the dimension of its arterioles by the process of autoregulation. The relationship between cardiac output (CO), blood pressure (BP) and systemic vascular resistance (SVR) is given by the formula:

$$SVR = \frac{\text{Mean arterial pressure} - \text{Mean right atrial pressure}}{\text{Cardiac output}}$$

On the other hand, patients with acute myocardial infarction, traumatic and cardiogenic shock are prone to low blood flows caused by the inability of the heart to pump enough blood through the body and, as cardiac output is the product of systemic vascular resistance and blood pressure, it follows that a patient may have a near normal blood pressure despite a low cardiac output, should the vascular resistance be increased.

It must be realised that in the clinical situation:

❑ The ECG is *no* guide to assessing cardiac output.
❑ Blood pressure may be grossly misleading as resistance may increase in the presence of a low output (in order to maintain normal blood pressures).
❑ The best clinical assessment is made by the measurement of urine output and temperature of the body extremities (hands and feet).
❑ For proper assessment however, discrete measurements of cardiac output by one of various means described in this chapter need to be made.
❑ Complete assessment of the cardiovascular system can only be made by the measurement of the following independent variables: *blood flow*, *blood pressure* and *blood volume*.

Thermodilution method The technique of the measurement of cardiac output by thermodilution was originally met with much scepticism as an accurate method of flow measurement. However it is now recognised as an accepted technique that compares favourably with other methods and is most usefully employed in critical care situations.

The method involves the introduction of a thermodilution *flow directed catheter* (Swan-Ganz) within the circulation and a bolus of cold liquid injected via the catheter, into the superior vena cava or right atrium, and the resultant blood temperature change detected downstream within the pulmonary artery.

The catheter consists of three lumens; one having an exit located at right atrial level used for injection of the cold liquid; one that is continuous to the distal orifice and a third that is used for inflation of the balloon. Some 4 cm proximal to the tip of the catheter and located on the exterior surface is a temperature detector known as a *"thermistor"*. This semi-conductor element acts as an electrical resistor that has a large temperature coefficient. This means that its electrical resistance dramatically changes when sub-

FIGURE 70

Three different types of
Flow Directed
thermodilution
catheters used for the
measurement of
Cardiac Output.
(Reproduced with kind
permission of Baxter
Health Care Corp.)

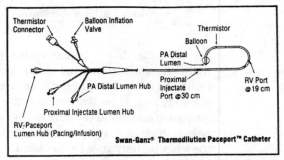

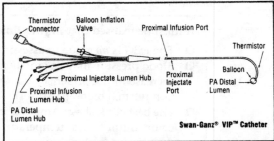

FIGURE 70

Three different types of
Flow Directed
thermodilution
catheters used for the
measurement of
Cardiac Output.
(Reproduced with kind
permission of Baxter
Health Care Corp.)

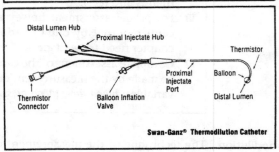

jected to changes in temperature (approximately 6.0 %/°C.) as compared to other resistor elements (0.4 %/°C).

Unfortunately, the relationship between resistance change and temperature is a non-linear one and necessitates the use of an electronic amplifier and computer to correct this characteristic and to calculate the area of the produced temperature/time curve.

Theory

Let us imagine a pipe having a flow of warm water through it at a constant rate and at some point we inject a bolus of ice cold liquid into the stream via a catheter within the pipe (Figure 71).

We could assume that the temperature of the water within the pipe as measured at some point downstream would be lowered by a specific amount (dF) depending upon:

A The temperature of the injected cold liquid.

B The volume of the injected cold liquid.

C The volume of water per unit time (flow) passing in the pipe between the site of injection and the point of measurement.

D The temperature of the water flowing in the pipe and

E Other factors such as thermal conductivity of the injectate catheter, injecting syringe etc.

In order to measure the flow of water (C) in the pipe, factors A, B, D and E would need to be known and the following equation for C determined.

$$C = \frac{B \times (A - B) \times E}{dF}$$

Now imagine a catheter that has been introduced into a vein and its tip advanced to the pulmonary artery; the catheter having an orifice at a point approximating the level of the right atrium through which an ice cold bolus of fluid can be injected. At the distal end of the catheter is located a thermistor that will measure temperature of the blood surrounding it.

Before the injection of a bolus of cold liquid of known temperature (A) and volume (B), the temperature of the blood (D) is determined i.e. body temperature. The temperature difference (dF) is determined by the thermistor attached to the wall of the catheter downstream to the site of injection. As the cold solution cools the blood that passes over the thermistor its electrical output will rise to a peak of coolness and fall exponentially and follow a temperature/time curve.

Thermal conductivity variants (E) i.e. the absorption of heat by the injectate catheter as the fluid passes through it, are minimal provided that the procedure is correctly performed and that the compensatory adjustments of the amplifier/computer are correctly set. There are other important factors that will minimally affect cardiac output measurement such as: cooling of the blood by the injectate that remains within the catheter; heat losses between the site of injection and detection; cyclic temperature changes within the right atrium, etc.

Connection of a recorder to the output of the computer will permit a temperature-time curve to be recorded which is in effect the linear relationship of the thermistor output after the injection of the ice cold bolus into the right atrium. The curve presented on the recording device would be seen as a sharp rise (as the temperature of the blood cools) that will peak at the maximal temperature change and gradually fall in an exponential manner to the baseline. The area within this calibrated curve is proportional to the cardiac output.

$$CO = \frac{V \times (Tb - Ti)}{a} \times \frac{Si - Ci}{Sb \times Cb} \times \frac{60 \times Ct \times K}{1}$$

where:

CO = cardiac output (ℓ/min)

V = injectate volume

A = area of curve (mm²)

Tb, Ti = temperature of blood and injectate

Sb, Si = specific gravity of blood and injectate

Cb, Ci = specific heat of blood and injectate

Ct = correction factor for injectate warming

K = calibration factor (mm/degrees C)

60 = 60 s/min

Since $\dfrac{Si \times Ci}{Sb \times Cb}$ = 1.08

when 5 % dextrose is used as the injectate. Asimplified form of this equation related to A, B, C, D and E (figure 71) may be constructed as:

$$CO = \frac{B \times (D - A) \times 1.08 \times 60}{\text{Area under curve}}$$

where 1.08 is a correction factor (E).

FIGURE 71

The principle of thermal dilution (see text)

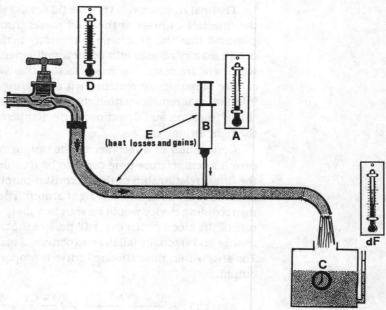

Technique

Operation of the cardiac output computer to which the thermodilution catheter is attached will depend on the model used and the operator must first familiarise himself with the instructions supplied. Control settings must be adjusted according to the model and type of catheter connected. Most units have the ability to check the thermistor integrity in vitro.

Prior to the study it is important that several samples of the injectate contained in end-capped plastic syringes are immersed in an ice bath for a period of at least 30 min to allow for equilibration. A separate water-filled end-capped syringe without the plunger that contains a temperature probe or an expanded thermometer is also immersed in the bath. Once the computer has been calibrated and all settings adjusted (if not automatically accepted by the computer) that relate to injectate volume, blood and injectate temperature etc., injection of the cold liquid may be performed. Removal of the end stop and transfer of the syringe to the Luer female fitting of the catheter should be carried out as rapidly as possible and the injection should take place as soon as the computer settings have been established. It is important that handling of the injectate syringe be minimised prior to injection to avoid a temperature rise of the injectate. Injection must be rapid in order to create the required bolus.

The use of a plastic coiled tube that is immersed in a beaker of ice cold water, from which the samples of injectate can be withdrawn when required does obviate the problems associated with syringe handling as described above.

Because of thermal losses within the lumen of the catheter, this first recorded output is always unreliable and should be repeated as soon as possible. It has been recommended by some workers that the residual injectate be withdrawn immediately after the injection is completed. This has the disadvantage of warming the inner lumen of the catheter. It is better to perform the second and subsequent studies as quickly as possible before the catheter has time to warm. It must be remembered that accurate cardiac output can only be achieved if the complete volume of the cold injectate is liberated from the end of the catheter and not allowed to mix with residual blood or injectate contained within its lumen.

Problems

Because certain manufacturers recommend that specific catheters be used with their equipment it is important that they be compatible although most computers will allow "foreign" catheters to be used provided that the controls are manually preset. Some of the problems associated with failure to obtain an expected output may be attributed to careless handling of the injectate and/or improper injection. Poor siting of the thermistor which may not be free within the pulmonary artery e.g. lying against the vessel wall, may cause permanent or intermittent loss of measurements.

The method of thermodilution as a means of measurement of cardiac output has obvious limitations and cannot be compared to the advantages of the multiple uses of dye dilution studies, but it does not require arterial puncture and can be performed with comparable ease at the bedside where rapid serial studies are required. The accuracy of the method when correctly performed qualifies it to be a useful diagnostic technique.

Troubleshooting

Problem	Cause	Solution
Cardiac output measurements too inaccurate, or absent	• Thermistor poorly sited	• Withdraw and re-insert
	• Incompatible catheter used	• Replace
	• Poor technique	• q.v. Problems
	• Due to pathology	• Check
	• Damage to thermistor	• Replace

The Fick method Determination of cardiac output by the Fick method is still considered by some investigators as a yardstick of measurement and although the method had, for many years, been in use in catheterisation laboratories throughout the world it is a time consuming technique that has recently lost much favour.

The principle is as follows:

1. The amount of oxygen absorbed during normal resting ventilation is calculated.
2. Blood withdrawn from sites in the circulation prior to it entering and after leaving the lungs is analysed for oxygen content.

In the normal intact heart the pulmonary blood flow must equal the cardiac output and from 1 and 2 above the cardiac output may be calculated from the formula:

$$\text{Cardiac output (CO)} = \frac{\text{Oxygen consumption} \times 100}{a\text{-}v \ O_2 \text{ difference}}$$

where oxygen consumption is measured in ml/min, and the a-v O_2 difference represents the difference of oxygen content of the two blood samples in volumes per cent.

Technique

Cardiac output is usually determined during the procedure of cardiac catheterisation when a catheter is passed into the pulmonary artery. This vessel is preferred to either of the great vessels entering the right heart or the chambers because of the normal differences in oxygen content of the inferior and superior vena cava. (In the adult, the SVC is usually lower in oxygen content than the IVC, whereas in the infant the SVC is higher than the IVC due to the smaller oxygen demand from the brain). Adequate mixing therefore of the SVC and IVC does not occur prior to the pulmonary artery. A needle or cannulae is also introduced into a superficial artery.

The patient's expired air is collected in a *Douglas bag* for a period of not less than five minutes, during which time blood samples are withdrawn simultaneously from the pulmonary artery and superficial artery into syringes that have been previously lubricated with silicone and the dead space filled with heparin. Care must be taken not to introduce air bubbles during this procedure. Blood gas analysis should be carried out as quickly as possible after withdrawal. Should this not be possible the following technique should be observed:

After sampling a syringe cap or end stop must be filled with mercury and fixed to the nipple of the syringe, so affording a complete seal. The sealed blood syringe should then be placed on a rotating device prior to analysis. If such a device is not available the syringe should be gently rotated by hand for one minute. This is done to allow mixing of the heparin. A sample of the patients expired air is removed after several washings of the sampling syringe, and the volume of air within the bag measured.

The sampled air from the patient together with a sample of the room air is analysed for oxygen content and the difference between the two (i.e. inspired and expired) is calculated. Oxygen consumption will equal the inspired/expired volume per cent multiplied be the volume of air expired per unit time.

Example:

(a) Amount of air in bag after 5 min expiration= 30 l.

(b) Room air oxygen content (inspired)= 20.9 vols%

(c) Expired air oxygen content= 17 vols%

(d) Inspired/expired oxygen content difference= 3.9 vols%

$$O_2 \text{ consumption } = \frac{d \times \left[\dfrac{(a) \text{ above}}{5} \right]}{100}$$

$$= \frac{3.9 \times 6000}{100}$$

$$= 234 \text{ cm}^3 / \text{min}$$

Oxygen content of arterial sample= 19.0 vols%
Oxygen content of pulmonary artery sample= 15.5 vols %

$$\text{Cardiac output (CO)} = \frac{234}{19 - 15.5}$$

$$= 6.7 \text{ litres/min}$$

Echocardiography Cardiac output may be calculated by advanced computerised echocardiography machines provided that the necessary software has been incorporated. Its analysis provides approximate calculation of cardiac output by the product of stroke volume and heart rate.

$$CO = \frac{EDV - ESV}{1000} \times \frac{60}{RR}$$

where:

EDV = end diastolic volume

ESV = end systolic volume

RR = interval (ms)

and entails the calculation of dimensions that have been previously measured and stored within the computer. There are many available methods or rules of measurement of volume (cubed, single and bi-plane ellipse, Simpson, Bullet), the most commonly used is the modified rule of Simpson.

Simpson's method of calculating area is shown in figure 72. By dividing the area into equal strips and measurements taken of the distances they are apart and their lengths, the area may be calculated. A modified version of calculations taken in more than one plane will allow approximate volume to be measured. In practice it entails the measurement of many area dimensions taken from:

❑ the LV area at the level of the mitral valve at end diastole and end systole (LVAMD, LVESD).

❑ the LV area at the level of the papillary muscle at and diastole and end systole (LVAPD, LVAPS).

❑ the LV long axis dimension at end of diastole and end systole (LVLD, LVLS).

Figure 72 is an example of Simpson's rule of measurement of area showing, (A) the apical long axis 2-chamber view of the left atrium and ventricle as mesured during diastole and systole. The projected chamber view of the ventricle (B) shows the sub divisions, $2n$ of equal parts. The ordinates are shown as $y_1, y_2, y_3 . y_2 n+1$ respectively. The Area = 1/3 AP (sum of the 1st and last ordinates + 2 × the sum of the other odd ordinates + 4 × the sum of the even ordinates.

FIGURE 72

The Echocardiographical measurement of cardiac output

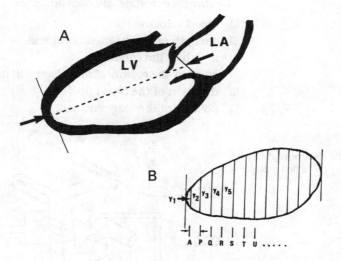

Other less common methods of measurement

A method of relative measurement of cardiac output was originally described by Kubicek et al[40] by the use of an *impedance cardiograph*. Four metal band electrodes are situated in pairs around the neck and mid thoracic areas of the patient. The two outer electrodes are connected to a high-frequency generator that permits a 100 000 Hz frequency to enter the body. The two inner electrodes receive the impedance changes of the thorax caused by increasing and decreasing amounts of blood within the thorax during each phase of the cardiac cycle. The output is recorded as electrical impedance changes that are similar in contour to the normal peripheral arterial pulse. The apparatus provides a first derivative output which, when recorded with an electrocardiogram and a phonocardiogram will provide indirect information of the cardiac function and output. Such a method causes minimal discomfort to the patient and the instrument is simple to use. It is not truly quantative but is capable of detecting small variations of thoracic blood flow.

The *electromagnetic flowmeter* is an instrument that will quantitatively measure the volumetric rate of blood flow by electromagnetic means. It does this by the use of a simple and fundamental magnetic principle, based on the induction of an electromagnetic force (EMF), or voltage, in a conductor moving within a magnetic field. Faraday's law of electro-magnetic induction informs us that the EMF is induced at right angles to the magnetic field and the direction of motion of the conductor. Blood, being an electrical conductor will produce a voltage relative to its mean velocity of motion within the magnetic field.

The *strength of voltage* will depend upon:

- blood velocity
- strength of the magnetic field and
- length of the conductor
  whereas the *polarity of the voltage* will depend upon the:
- direction of the blood flow and
- polarity of the magnetic field.

FIGURE 73

The electromagnetic
flowmeter

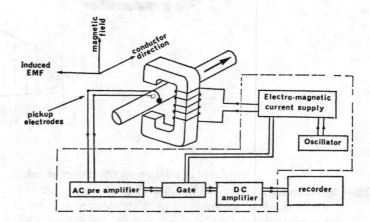

Note the inset depicting the thumb rule of Flemming in the upper left corner

Figure 73 shows a conductor situated within the poles of a magnet and the "thumb rule" of Fleming illustrating how the induced current is measured in relation to the magnetic field and direction of conduction, or blood flow. The induced EMF that is sensed by the electrodes in contact with the outer surface of the blood vessel is electronically amplified. The poles of the small electro-magnet situated on diagonally opposite sides of the blood vessel are magnetised by the passing of a current through coils that surround them. Both the poles and the pickup electrodes are usually encased within a plastic resin material in the shape of an incomplete circle. This portion of the instrument is known as the *probe* or *transducer* and is positioned around the vessel in which flow measurement is required. Connected to the probe is an insulated cable that contains both energising and pickup conductive wires that connect to the control unit.

Electromagnetic flowmeters are usually identified by the wave shape of the energizing signal that produces the magnetic field in the probe, i.e. square, trapezoidal, sinusoidal or direct current. Calibration and sensitivity of the instrument is performed by means of an integrator circuit incorporated within the control unit. It does this by summation of the blood volume passing through the probe dependent on the sensitivity and independent of the flow rate. It is extremely important that the probe used for blood flow measurement is a good snug fit around the vessel. For this reason many types and sizes of probes are often required.

The electromagnetic flow meter has many applications in surgery of the heart, great vessels and in the field of reconstructive surgery and many advantages over other methods of blood flow measurement:

1. Instantaneous blood flow readings are obtained in ccs/minute.
2. It is able to differentiate forward from backward flow.
3. Viscosity, temperature and pressure of the blood contained within the vessel does not affect calibration.
4. It does not necessitate the opening of the blood vessel and therefore obviating the risks associated with direct puncture of an artery. It does not of course obviate the need to expose the vessel.

Catheter-tipped electromagnetic flow meters are also used that may be inserted within the vessel.

Many other methods of measuring cardiac output have been described[41, 42, 43, 44] that are either empirical, inaccurate or not clinically suitable.

Further reading Carr JJ & Brown JM. *Introduction to Biomedical Equipment Technology.* Prentice Hall 1993.

4 *The Intra-Aortic Balloon Pump*

A major advancement occurred in 1967, during the year of the world's first heart transplant, when Kantrowitz and co-workers[45] clinically applied intra-aortic balloon counterpulsation for the treatment of patients with myocardial infarction refractory to medical therapy.

The act of inflating and deflating a balloon located within the thoracic aorta has today become an accepted therapeutic technique for the control of a variety of medical and surgical disorders:

❑ *Cardiogenic shock* This potentially irreversible condition commonly classified as *pump failure* occurs when the left ventricle is incapable of maintaining a cardiac output adequate for perfusion of the vital organs. It is associated with an acute and extensive myocardial dysfunction that reduces stroke volume and cardiac output and generally responds well to IABP therapy, although prognosis is directly related to the extent of necrosis. Other pump failure conditions may occur during:

   septic shock, chest trauma, intra-operative MI or post surgery.

❑ *Post infarction VSD* is a ventricular septal defect that occurs after an extensive infarction of the septum, the additional burden of the large left to right ventricular shunt severely compromising both right and left ventricles. The pulmonary blood flow is greatly increased, LV stroke output falls and systemic vaso-constriction is increased that causes an increase in afterload. This extra load that the LV cannot handle causes more blood to be diverted from left to right through the septum, so worsening left ventricular failure (LVEDP). Response to IABP is initially good and if surgery is not performed the patient may require counterpulsation for prolonged periods. Other post-infarction mechanical defects include: Ventricular aneurysms and severe papillary muscle dysfunction.

❑ *Unstable angina* may be classified as either pre- or postinfarction. Pre-infarction angina may present itself as 'stable' when a single coronary artery is obstructed and an adequate collateral circulation is present; or as 'unstable' when multi-vessel disease is present, spasm, or on-going thromboses producing repeated episodes of pain which may or may not be severe. The response to IABP therapy in this group of patients is usually excellent. Angina stops immediately and LVEDP is reduced.

FIGURE 74

The monitor panel of the Kontron KAAT 11 Intra Aortic Balloon Pump. The Inflation and Deflation controls are located at the right and left sides of the monitor scope.

Reproduced with kind permission of Arrow Africa Ltd.

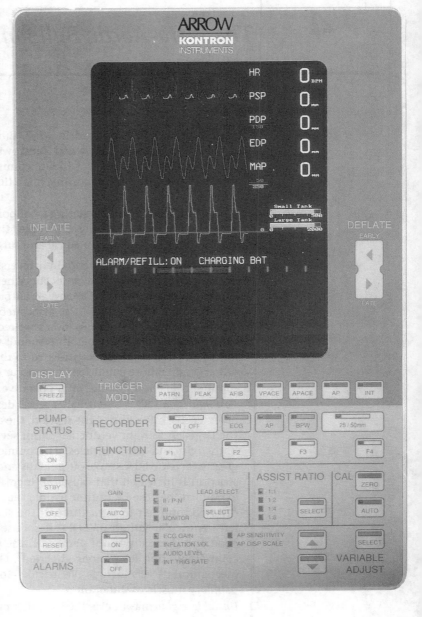

❑ *Ischemic related ventricular arrhythmias* are often corrected after the increased perfusion that intra-aortic balloon pumping affords.

❑ *Weaning off by-pass.* Patients having undergone cardiopulmonary by-pass may experience 'pump failure' and require assistance with an IABP when weaning off a heart-lung machine. Lengthy open heart procedures associated with periods of ischemia and heart incisions often cause depression of the myocardium which is unable to offer adequate circulatory support. IAPB therapy often affords the required support in this condition.

❑ *Peri-operative support* Such indications may include:
  • The containment of an area of injury, especially during an acute anterior infarction.
  • Prophylactic support of an ischemic patient during anaesthesia induction or cardiac catheterisation procedures that may include coronary angiography, PTCA or thrombolysis.
  • High risk patients that are subjected to cardiac or general surgery.

THEORY

To understand the principles of intra-aortic balloon pumping and to be able to afford the patient the maximum benefits it is of the utmost importance that a sound knowledge of basic cardiac physiology be known..

It is important that the meanings of such terminology as:
❑ balloon pressure waveform,
❑ isovolumetric contraction,
❑ perfusion,
❑ preload,
❑ afterload, and
❑ contractility

are fully understood and how each one is affected by intra-aortic balloon pumping

---

Let us first consider what benefits the patient may expect when a balloon of some 40 cc's volume and 20 mm diameter is inserted into the descending thoracic aorta and is caused to inflate during ventricular diastole and deflate during systole.

Three major changes take place. There is

1. An *increase* in coronary perfusion pressure

2. A *decrease* in preload and afterload and

3. A *decrease* in myocardial oxygen demand

FIGURE 75
The physiological
mechanisms of the left
side of the heart

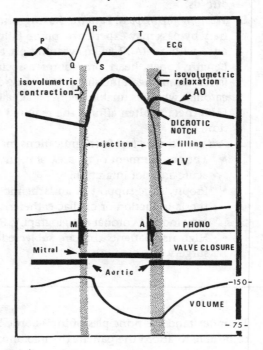

Let us now consider the mechanisms by which intra-aortic balloon pumping can create these changes:

1. The *flow* of oxygenated blood through the coronary vasculature is, within limits, directly related to the applied *pressure*, provided the *resistance* is constant i.e. the higher the pressure within the aorta the greater the flow and, conversely, the lower the pressure the lesser the flow. Inversely, flow is related to the coronary vascular resistance. The higher the resistance, the lesser the flow. The lesser the resistance, the greater the flow, provided the pressure is constant. These are general rules, but of course the resistance of the coronary vasculature constantly varies as the heart contracts and relaxes, as does the pressure. During systole when the heart has contracted the resistance of the coronary vasculature is high. As blood is ejected forcibly and rapidly from the left ventricular chamber, most of it by-passes the ostia and little enters. It is during *diastole* that the heart musculature receives most of its blood, for it is then that the coronary vascular resistance is minimal.

By inflating the balloon that lies within the aorta during diastole, the passage of blood to the lower extremities ceases until such time as the balloon deflates and the aortic valve opens during the systolic phase. This period of inflation of the balloon increases the diastolic pressure within the ascending aorta and its tributaries, so allowing a greater flow of blood through the coronary arteries. It is this increase of diastolic pressure that is known as *diastolic augmentation*.

2. Now imagine the left ventricle during *systole*. The excitation impulse has spread through the myocardium from the apex to the base. The pressure within the ventricle rapidly increases as the myocardium forcibly contracts against the closed mitral and aortic valves. This period, known as *isovolumetric contraction*, is the time taken for the ventricle to build up enough pressure in order to open the aortic valve, i.e. the diastolic pressure within the aorta. It is during this period that the work of the heart and its oxygen demand is greatest. The higher the diastolic pressure the greater the amount of work it has to generate *(afterload)* in order to force the blood through the valve.

Now imagine the balloon to deflate as systole commences. Where there was an inflated balloon occupying the descending thoracic aorta, there is suddenly a vacuum i.e. an empty space of 40 cc's volume which has the effect of increasing the momentum of the ejected blood within the root of the aorta. It is this sudden decrease in volume that lowers the resistance, and therefore the work or afterload, that the LV has to overcome. The LV volume prior to ejection i.e. the end diastolic myocardial fibre length, commonly known as the *preload* is also greatly reduced.

3. The heart muscle normally consumes approximately 75 % of the total oxygen content of the arterial blood that enters the coronary arteries. The venous desaturated blood returns to the right atrium via

   (*a*) the coronary sinus, which accounts for some 60 % of the total volume of venous drainage, and

   (*b*) the anterior coronary vein and

   (*c*) the remainder draining into both the right atrium and ventricle via the many small veins that enter these chambers.

   Because of the high oxygen demand of the heart the oxygen saturation of the returning myocardial blood is extremely low, presenting a large arterial/ venous difference.

During the isovolumetric contraction phase the heart utilises approximating 90 % of its total oxygen requirement during the entire cardiac cycle. Such is the energy expended by the myocardium in order to create the pressure to open the aortic valve.

The act of *inflating* the balloon during diastole changes the whole haemodynamic scene,[46] e.g:

❑ The aortic pressure is increased and therefore the coronary blood flow to narrowed arteries and collateral vessels is improved

❑ Left ventricular compliance is improved and function enhanced, as seen by a reduction in both end diastolic and end systolic areas and also regional ejection fractions are considerably improved.

❑ The LVEDP is lowered which in turn enhances subendocardial perfusion and myocardial oxygen supply[47]

❑ There is a decrease of the radius of the LV producing lessening of wall tension and subsequent decrease in myocardial oxygen demand (MVO_2)

❑ Because of a decrease in the filling pressure of the left heart there is also an improved right ventricular performance[48]

❑ There is a slight improvement of systemic perfusion believed to be caused by increased ventricular ejection that is directly related to the elasticity of the aortic wall.[49]

Figure 76A shows inflation commencing at closure of the aortic valve and ending pre systole. Notice the augmentation of diastolic pressure (increasing coronary perfusion) and the decrease of aortic end diastolic pressure (reducing myocardial oxygen demand). The initial pulse contour and the dotted lines represent the non-assisted aortic pressure.

FIGURE 76 A

The changes in aortic blood pressure after cyclic balloon deflation and inflation (see text)

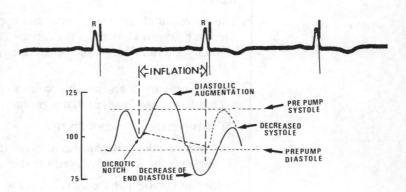

It should be realised that not all patients will obtain the maximum benefits of intra-aortic balloon pumping. The amplitude of the augmented waveform may not be as tall as expected. Much depends upon physiological, pathological and pharmacological circumstances related to the patients condition. For example, Coronary perfusion may change little if the vessels are maximally dilated. Often, the IABP is used so late in the treatment of acute myocardial infarction that it is of minimum benefit to the acutely damaged and compromised heart. *Hypovolemic* and *hypertensive* patients often present a reduced augmentation. There are many technical factors that may prevent an adequate augmentation, i.e. Low balloon volume, too small balloon size, position of balloon too low in aorta , etc.

Patients with very low peripheral pressures often do not respond to counter-pulsation with balloon therapy unless combined with a pharmacological agent. Similarly, it cannot be expected to effectively reduce the myocardial workload if consideration is not given to the importance of balloon inflation and deflation in relation to the cardiac cycle. Ideally, the balloon should inflate at aortic valve closure and deflate at aortic valve opening. In stating this, one would believe that the 1st and 2nd heart sounds of mitral and aortic valve closure respectively would be the ideal triggering events for balloon pumping. Unfortunately it is technically difficult to time from heart sounds, due to the high amplification required and in general the instability of long term phonocardiograph recordings. Extraneous noises and the large variations of acoustic amplitude (signal to noise ratio) that often occur within the immediate work area would effect the operation of the pump mechanism. Pump timing is therefore triggered from the more stable ECG and/or arterial pressure.

The relatively high frequency component and amplitude of the R wave of the ECG make it an ideal triggering marker to deflate the balloon and the dichrotic notch of the arterial pressure wave to trigger inflation.

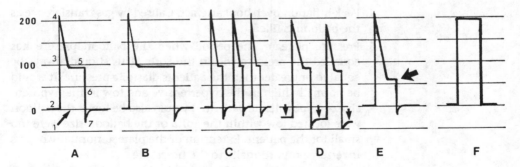

FIGURE 76B

Some BPW seen when counterpulsating. A — the components of the balloon pressure waveform illustrating its seven segments. B — bradycardia showing extension of the plateau. C — tachycardia. D — slow gas leak showing a gradual negative deviation of the baseline (arrows). E — Hypotensive (arrow shows a decreased plateau) and F — wrong size balloon used.

BALLOON PRESSURE WAVEFORM (BPW)

The waveform produced within the balloon is undoubtedly a very important one. It is a built-in 'trouble shooting' guide for the operator of the balloon pump who should soon realise that the pressure produced within the balloon and presented on the pump monitor has a distinct contour (Figure 76B). This contour has set limitations of normality and any variations of the waveform outside of normal limits should be immediately examined, an assessment made and the cause identified.

> *Note:* Abnormal balloon pressure waveforms may be due to faulty operation of the system and could be critical to the well-being of the patient.

The waveform consists of seven segments and abnormal deflections of any should receive immediate attention. (Figure 76B).

1. The fixed zero reference baseline of the monitor.
2. The balloon pressure baseline. The pressure level after deflation of the balloon. Usually not more than 2.5 mm Hg above the reference baseline. A fall below this baseline, would indicate either a low or high leak of helium gas from the system, depending whether the fall is gradual or rapid. The pressure plateau would also grdually decrease signifying a loss of pressure within the balloon.
3. Inflation rise. The start of the compression cycle signifying rapid gaseous inflation of the balloon. The steeper the vertical the slope the faster the inflation.
4. Peak inflation overshoot artefact. Caused by gas transference as the balloon is filled.
5. Pressure plateau. The period when the balloon presure has equalled the pressure within the aorta. This should always be equal to or greater than the patients diastolic pressure. It would be normally high in the hypertensive and low in the hypotensive or hypovolemic patient. It would also be low if the balloon were located low within the aorta or the balloon size were too small for the patient. Extension of the plateau normally occurs inversely proportionally to the heart rate.
6. Deflation fall. The end of the compression cycle indicating the rapid decrease of gaseous pressure as the helium is exhausted from the balloon.
7. Peak deflation overshoot artefact. Caused by the resistance of the catheter as the gas is transferred from the balloon.

Normal variations of this waveform will be seen when there are changes in the heart rate, cardiac cycle or blood pressure.

Abnormal variations may be due to:

❑ Incorrect balloon size (figure 76, segments 4, 5, & 7).
❑ Extreme late deflation (7)
❑ Loss of helium gas, either internal within the pump or external in the connecting tubing or balloon catheter. (2 and 5)
❑ Poor transmission of gas caused by either partial or severe obstruction of gas to and/or from the balloon. The width of the waveform is increased. (3–6), often caused after insertion of a balloon in a tortuous vessel or by a partial kink where the catheter enters the groin. Check whether the plateau (5) is high with a loss of the peak artefact (4). Look for the cause of obstruction.

Ask:

❑ Is the balloon too high or too low within the aorta?
❑ Is the balloon completely unwrapped?
❑ Is the balloon too large for the patient?
❑ Is the balloon within the intimal wall of the artery?

Note: The technologist or nurse should *not* undertake the responsibilities of intra-aortic balloon pumping unless fully conversant with the interpretation of the balloon pressure wave abnormalities. They not only inform the operator of the systems function but are the only waveforms that give the information that will allow the operator to correct any problems he or she may encounter. Memorise the balloon pressure waveform changes that you would expect when there is:

❑ Hypertension
❑ Hypotension or Hypovolemia
❑ Bradycardia
❑ Tachycardia
❑ Arrhythmias
❑ A small helium gas loss
❑ A large helium gas loss
❑ A helium gas obstruction
❑ Kinks in the catheter line or balloon
❑ Wrong size balloon inserted

Know what to do in the event of a power failure. It may be unwise to leave the ballon within the aorta for prolonged periods.

Learn how to wean your patient off the pump. This may entail reducing the balloon pressure and/or reducing the frequency of pumping. The technologist should consult the cardiologist or surgeon before this manouvre is carried out.

For more detailed information regarding function and management of your particular machine, consult the Information Manual that was delivered with your pump or, your representative.

Recent advanced technology has today made available semi-portable machines weighing less than 30 kg are able to trigger via radio frequency transmission; use non-sheath balloons; have more reliable sensing and triggering algorithms; improved monitoring facilities and some that will allow extremely rapid inflation and deflation timing to rates of 170 bpm at full volume displacement.

Further reading

❑ Quaal SJ, *Comprehensive intra-aortic balloon pumping*. CV Mosby Company. St. Louis, Missouri. 1984.

❑ Bregman D, Haubert SM, Self MA: Intra-aortic balloon counter-pulsation *A primr. J.Cardiovasc. Med*: 9, No.8, 607,1984.

❑ *Physiology and principles of counterpulsation*. Arrow/Kontron Training Manual, 1994.

❑ *Seminar for Intra-Aortic Balloon Pumping*. Datascope Clinical Evaluation Services. Datascope Corp., Montvale, NJ. USA.

5   *Electronic Pacing of the Heart*

THE ELECTRONIC PACEMAKER

The artificial cardiac pacemaker is an electronic *generator* that discharges repetitive electrical impulses to the heart via one or two wire *electrodes*. Its purpose is to substitute for the physiological pacemakers of the heart.

The first implantation of a cardiac pacemaker designed by Dr R. Elmqvist, was performed by Dr Ake Senning at the Karolinska Hospital at Stockholm, Sweden in 1958. These early pacemakers were bulky devices (±70 grams), used traditional bi-polar transistor discrete technology consisting of a few resistors and capacitors and less than 10 transistors. They consumed so much power (milliamperes) from their mercury zinc batteries that they had a life of only three to less than nine months. They were 'fixed rate' devices, meaning that they discharged their impulses regardlessly until end of battery life or removal. Later models used integrated film circuits in which the components were built into a glass substrate which allowed an extension of life to a few years. The film module together with the mercury batteries was encapsulated in epoxy resin.

The pacemaker of today is an engineering masterpiece by comparison. It uses VLSI (Very Large Scale Integration) CMOS (Complementary Metal Oxide Semiconductors) 1 µm circuitry technology comprising several thousand transistors, drains approximately 20 µA of current, weighs 20–40 grams, and its lithium composite battery has a longevity of 5 to 15 years, depending upon the complexity of the design, the frequency it is used and its preset performance parameters.

There are three major components of the *pacemaker system:*

1. The *power source,* or battery, that is used to supply the necessary power.
2. The *electronic circuitry,* that 1. generates the required timing impulses to be transmitted to the heart and 2. senses incoming signals delivered from the heart.
3. The *electrode* or electrodes, commonly known as the lead/s transmit the impulses to and from the surface of the heart.

The power source and the electronic circuitry are contained in a single hermetically sealed metal case (titanium or stainless steel) known as the pacemaker or generator.

FIGURE 77
The three major components of the pacemaker system

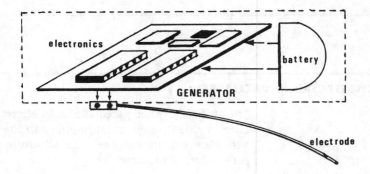

Before we go further, let us discuss some fundamentals of a pacemaker system. The purpose of the pacemaker is to provide sufficient electrical energy to the heart. The electrode, when connected to the pacemaker and its distal tip located against the wall either within or without the heart chamber, provides the electrical communication to cause that chamber to depolarise and contract. Imagine an electrode that has been introduced into a branch of the cephalic vein and the distal tip to be in contact with the endocardial surface of the right ventricle (where most ventricular electrodes are positioned). Imagine too that the pacemaker is implanted within the right pectoralis fascia (a common site of implantation). The electrode siting would be *endocardial* and the location of the pacemaker in the *right pectoral* region.

Physiologically the two lower chambers of the heart are electrically connected, as are the two upper chambers, so that when an electrical impulse transmitted via the electrode, reaches the endocardial surface of the right ventricle, the chamber will depolarise and subsequently spread its excitation across the septal and myocardial fibres to cause the left ventricle to depolarise. The electrocardiograph pattern will be very similar to a left bundle branch block *(LBBB)*, a situation when the right ventricle is depolarised before the left. The QRS complex will be wide and there will be a pacemaker artefact or 'spike' preceding the QRS complex (Figure 78). The spike is the discharge impulse from the pacemaker and, when followed by a QRS complex, indicates that the pacemaker has 'captured' or depolarised the chamber. Failure to capture the heart would be seen as a pacemaker spike that is *not* followed by a QRS complex as seen in figure 79.

FIGURE 78
The normal pacemaker
electrogram showing
the impulse or 'spike'
that precedes the wid-
ened QRS complex.

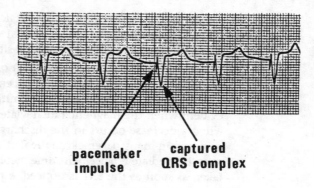

pacemaker
impulse

captured
QRS complex

FIGURE 78
The normal pacemaker
electrogram showing
the impulse or 'spike'
that precedes the wid-
ened QRS complex.

FIGURE 79
An impulse that is not
followed by a QRS com-
plex and therefore does
not cause depolarisa-
tion ot the chamber.

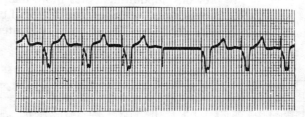

THE PACEMAKER BATTERY

Many power sources have been used since the first pacemaker was implanted and have included mercury cells; nickel-cadmium rechargeable cells, radioactive isotopes (Plutonium Pu-238 activating thermopiles or Promethium Pm-149 operating a beta-voltaic battery) and, since the development of the lithium-iodine electrochemical system in 1969 by Catalyst Research Corporation, several types of lithium composites, all using lithium metal as the anode for the cell. These include lithium/silverchromate, lithium/lead iodide, lithium/thionyl chloride, and lithium/cupricsulphide. Although the performance characteristics of each kind may vary they are all capable of delivery of comparatively high, stable voltages at low current levels. The most commonly used and reliable is the lithium-iodine, a battery that complies favourably with engineering specifications as the ideal pacemaker power source.[50] Unlike the other lithium cells, it has no liquid electrolyte and therefore no gas is given off by the cell and it does not require a separator to avoid contact between the anode and the cathode.

The point of cell depletion or *end of life* (EOL) is the time at which useful life of the power cell is ended and is usually defined by cell manufacturers as the time when the open circuit voltage drops to a predetermined value, after which a rapid decline can be expected.

The indications of approaching EOL vary with each pacemaker manufacturer and are commonly related to the rate of discharge when a magnet is positioned over the site of the implanted device.

The *elective replacement time* (ERT) or *recommended replacement time* (RRT) is the time when the pacemaker can be comfortably removed from the body within a limited time, and will become evident when the magnetic rate deviates from indicated levels, or when a decrease occurs in the discharge rate. Two indicators are common in many pacemakers: the first as an elective and a second as an immediate replacement time. Replacement should be undertaken as soon as the ERT is noticed, especially when the patients previous appointment was more than a few months ago. Many programmers will allow the degree of battery depletion to be also verified on an LCD, printer or computer screen.

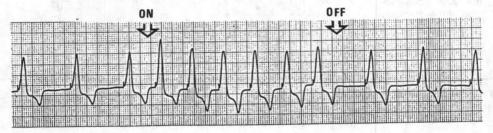

FIGURE 80

A common indicator of battery status after placement of a magnet over the pacemaker site. The discharge rate is caused to increase to a specific value. A decrease is indicative of a low battery charge.

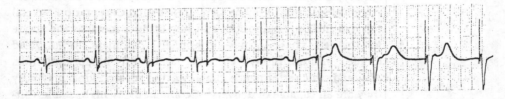

FIGURE 81

Determination of battery status of a patient in sinus rhythm at a rate higher than the preset pacing rate. The impulses can be clearly seen to invade the rhythm until it becomes possible for capture to occur, i.e. outside the refractory period.

Battery depletion may not be the only reason for surgical removal or replacement of the pacemaker. It may be necessary for a variety of *medical* reasons such as:

❑ sepsis,

❑ pacemaker syndrome,

❑ erosion of the electrode or generator through the skin,

❑ discomfort,

❑ to provide greater physiological benefit to the patient, etc,

or for *technical* reasons, such as:

❑ circuitry malfunction,

❑ intermittent electrical connection of the electrode,

❑ electrode displacement within heart chamber,

❑ damage by electromagnetic interference (EMI), etc.

Although the *technical* reasons above are uncommon and/or often preventable, battery current drain may also be due to:

❑ lead fracture,

❑ dislodgement of the electrode tip ,

❑ breakage of electrode insulation,

Often, the presence of abnormal threshold readings will give an indication of the fault.

❑ High voltage, low current, therefore high impedance — suspect electrode fracture

❑ High voltage, high current, therefore normal impedance — suspect dislodgement.

❑ Low voltage, high current, therefore low impedance — possible insulation defect

NBG GENERIC PACEMAKER CODE

To help understand the function of a particular pacemaker it is obviously important that certain technical characteristics be known. Until a mere decade ago, many who were associated with pacing technology were still using cumbersome and lengthy definitions to describe the function of an implanted device. It was because of the increasing complexity of pacemakers that the Intersociety Commission on Heart Disease Resources *(ICHD)* developed a three letter code that was intended to simplify understanding of the operation and function of a pacemaker. This code was revised to a five letter system in order to accommodate later programming and anti-tachyarrhythmia features.

In 1987 the North American Society for Pacing and Electrophysiology (NASPE) and the British Pacing and Electrophysiology Group (BPEG) compiled a new code that would be more acceptable to further advances in pacing and also defibrillatory technology. This code was to be known as the *NASPE/BPEG generic pacemaker code* or, in its abbreviated form, the *NBG code*,[51] and like the ICHD code is represented by five positions that are designated by Roman numerals.

The first position designates the *chamber paced* and contains one of four letters — O, A, V, D.

O = None
A = Atrium
V = Ventricle
D = Dual (A + V)

These letters refer to the chamber to which the distal portion of the electrode is attached in order to pace that chamber. It may either be in contact with the endocardial, myocardial or epicardial portion or surface of either of the atria or ventricles, i.e. the chamber(s) to which the electrical impulses from the pacemaker are transmitted. This may be the Atrium (A), Ventricle (V), or it may be a Dual system (D) where one electrode is located in the Atrium and the other in the Ventricle or there is no pacing of either chamber (O).

The second position refers to the *chamber sensed:*

O = None
A = Atrium
V = Ventricle
D = Dual (A + V)

It denotes the chamber from which the hearts own electrical activity is sensed by the pacemaker. This may be the Atrium (A), Ventricle (V), both Atrium and Ventricle (D) or none at all (O). Like the first position it refers only to anti-bradyarrhythmia function. In a single electrode system the pacing and sensing chambers are usually the same.

The third position is the *response to sensing:*

O = None
I = Inhibited
T = Triggered
D = Dual (A + V)

It tells us how the pacemaker will respond to sensing of signals that originate from the heart. It may withhold or *inhibit (I)* the discharge of an impulse until a certain period has passed and then resume its discharge, or it may, on sensing a signal from the heart, discharge an impulse. In other words the discharge of the impulse is *triggered (T)* from the signal it senses. Also, the pacemaker may allow *dual (D)* modes of action i.e. it may inhibit and trigger, or it may not respond at all (O).

Figure 82 details the function of a DVO pacemaker and although not an accepted mode of operation it does help to better undersatand the meaning of the escape intervals.

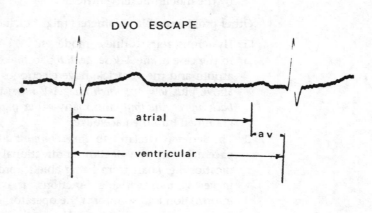

FIGURE 82
The escape intervals of a DVO pacemaker which can pace both atrial and ventricular chambers and sense only the ventricle. Should a ventricular response NOT occur within the atrial escape interval, the unit will discgarge to the atrium. Should this atrial discharge NOT cause a ventricular response, the pacemaker will discharge to the ventricle. The pre-programmed intervals will determine the A-V interval.

The fourth position (IV), the *programmability/rate adaptiveness*:

O = None

P = Simple Programmable (less common)

M = Multiprogrammable

C = Communicative

R = Rate adaptiveness (or Modulation)

This gives information of the way in which the pacemaker is programmed (programmability) and whether its rate is controlled by some physiological or metabolic function (rate adaptiveness).

The pacemaker may be a *simple programmable* type, designated by the letter (P) that will allow the operator to adjust, with the aid of an external programmer, two electrical parameters, usually:

1. the *rate* of discharge of the impulse and
2. the *duration* or width of the electrical impulse, although many simple programmable types may include *sensitivity*.

Or should the pacemaker have more than two programmable functions it is generally known as a *multi-programmable* device designated by the letter (M). This means that apart from rate and pulse width it may also permit such functions to be programmed as:

❑ *Output*: The amplitude of the voltage that is delivered to the distal portion of the electrode.

❑ *Sensitivity*: The degree to which the pacemaker is able to respond to an extraneous signal. One can readily imagine that in order to sense the small amplitude signals that are delivered by the atrium, the pacemaker would require a much greater 'sensitivity' than were it required to detect, for example, the comparatively enormous amplitude signals that are delivered by the much thicker ventricle.

Other programmable parameters might include:

❏ Hysteresis, refractoriness, mode, etc.

❏ In the case of the *A-V sequential* pacemaker (to which both the atrium and the ventricle have electrodes attached), all of the above plus *low rate, high rate, A-V interval, ratesmoothing, fallback, upper rate limit* and many other parameters may be programmed into the pacemaker.

❏ The letter (C) relates to the *communicative* properties of the pacemaker which will allow bi-directional telemetered communication i.e. apart from being able to program into the pacemaker various variable functions, it can also retrieve the information and so inform the operator as to how it has been programmed. This is achieved by placing a hand-held programmer over the pacemaker area and initiating a response, information of which may be read from a LCD screen or paper printer.

Most pacemakers with bi-directional capabilities will also allow the operator to transmit into the pacemaker such information as:

❏ Date of and the reasons for implantation.

❏ Electrical threshold and impedance values at the time of implantation.

❏ Measured P or R wave amplitudes.

❏ Type and model of implanted electrode(s).

❏ Medical information concerning the medication that the patient is taking.

❏ The pacemaker may also be programmed to allow the operator to retrieve information of the frequency of its discharge.

All of the preprogrammed data can be transmitted out of the pacemaker at any time during its life by a second operator who is in possession of a similar programmer. Many units will permit the transmission and recording of the electrogram *from* the electrode/heart interface. The letter (C) also tells us that the pacemaker is multi-programmable.

Figure 83 simply illustrates how, by placing a programmer over the site of the implanted generator allows the operator to transmit or receive data to or from the pacemaker. Changing of the many parameters, and individual segments of each parameter, is carried out by the transmission of pulsed radio frequency signals. For example, let us assume that a pacemaker is preprogrammed at a rate of 60 beats per minute, represented by a pulsed signal of 'f' Hz., that bursts for 't' ms at a period of 'p' ms that lasts for 'L' seconds duration. With such an enormous variety of timing combinations it is not surprising to realise how many parameters and segments within each parameter can be controlled. A change of frequency by a few cycles may change the rate by a few beats whilst programming a change in 't' or 'p' may allow change of refractory, pulse width, sensitivity or any of the many programmable function of that particular pacemaker.

FIGURE 83
Programming the co-municative pacemaker.

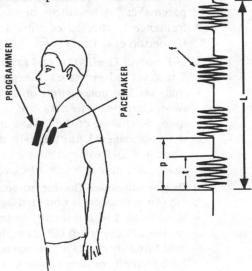

Rate adaptiveness Also known as rate responsiveness or rate modulation, the (R) of this code refers to the ability of the pacemaker to adapt its rate according to physiological and metabolic demands. Rate adaptive pacemakers may be VVI or DDD or a combination of either. It is therefore able to vary its rate by the use of bio-sensors that form part of the electrode/generator system allowing the pacemaker to vary its rate by sensing such physiologic variables as:

❏ *Minute ventilation* By emitting low energy pulses between the distal portion of the electrode and the generator the transthoracic impedance may be measured. With increase of respiratory rate on exercise the pacing rate is increased. One disadvantage of this system is that rate changes may occur relative to impedance changes that are not caused by exercise e.g. hyperventilation, sneezing, hiccoughs, coughing etc. (Rossi et al 1983)

❏ *Blood temperature* By the use of a thermistor located on the electrode, changes of the central venous blood temperature may be measured to cause the pacemaker rate to rise on exercise. Because the venous blood temperature drops at the onset of exercise and that low exercise produces little change in temperature, the sensitivity i.e. its capability to accurately measure changes of metabolic requirements, is poor. (Jolgren et al 1983)

❏ *Muscular activity* By the use of a piezoelectric crystal that is bonded to the inside of the metal can of the generator, muscular vibration around the area of the implanted pacemaker may be detected. This type of biosensor has the unique property of emitting minute electrical impulses when vibrated. In this instance the vibrations of muscle movement around the implanted area are sensed to cause an increase of rate of the pacemaker. The specificity or accuracy with which cardiac performance is affected of this bio-sensor is particularly poor. (Anderson et al 1986)

❑ *Q-T interval* The inverse and exponential relationship of the Q-T interval to heart rate is measured by the use of an electrode that has low polarisation qualities. By sensing the evoked T wave, changes in the period of pacemaker discharge and maximum downslope of the T wave are reflected as rate changes of the pacemaker. Unfortunately during steady state exercise, when the Q-T interval may not change, the pacemaker discharge rate may decrease. (Rickards & Norman 1983)

❑ *Oxygen saturation* The measurement of central venous blood oxygen saturation is obtained by the use of a dedicated electrode located within the right ventricle emitting red and infra-red light at every 4th QRS complex. The variation of reflected light intensity causes the pacemaker rate to vary proportionally. The specificity of such a biosensor is high. (Wirtzfeld et al 1987)

❑ *Stroke volume* Changes in stroke volume (dV/dT) are measured by impedance changes after the delivery of micro-pulses in the right ventricle. Systolic Time Intervals (STI) may also be measured by this type of biosensor. (Salo Olsen 1984)

❑ *RV pressure* This is accomplished by the use of a micro transducer that is located in the pacing electrode. This velocity device allows the rate of the pacemaker to change as the dP/dt changes during exercise. (Stangl 1987)

❑ *Acceleration* By the use of an accelerometer, body motion causes the rate to be increased. Because of a lower range of filtration and that the average output of the device is measured and not the vibration, the specificity and sensitivity of this sensor is higher when compared to other activity devices. (Alt et al 1989)

❑ *Blood pH* The use of a pH electrode sensor. Changes of blood acidity during exercise causes heart rate to increase. (Camilli et al 1983)

The letter O signifies no programmability or rate adaptiveness.
The fifth position (V) the *anti-tachyarrhythmia function*

O = None

P = Pacing (antitachy)

S = Shock

D = Dual (P + S)

The letter (P) or *pacing,* refers to the presence of one or more anti-tachyarrhythmia functions that will sense a rapid heart rate and automatically discharge a series of preprogrammed pacing impulses to a heart chamber in order to cease the tachyarrhythmia. The letter (S) or *shock* refers to the delivery of a defibrillatory impulse that is applied by means of an *Automatic Implanted Cardiovertor/Defibrillator (AICD)* device. The letter (D) would signify a pacemaker having anti-tachy and shock functions. (O) would indicate neither function present.

Let us now consider *how* this code is applied. The pacemaker that is most commonly implanted is the VVICO. This code informs us that:

❑ 1st letter. The chamber paced is the Ventricle (V),
❑ 2nd letter. The chamber sensed is also the Ventricle (V),
❑ 3rd letter. The pacemaker has the capability of being Inhibited (I) by any signal it senses,
❑ 4th letter. It has communicative functions (C) and,
❑ 5th letter. It has no anti-tachy function (O)
❑ Adding all five letters we have VVICO.

A DDDCP symbol informs us that the atrium *and* the ventricle (D = dual) have an electrode within them through which the impulses from the pacemaker are discharged. Both upper and lower chambers are being paced. From the second letter (D = dual) we know that through these two electrodes the pacemaker is able to sense any incoming signals from the atria and/or ventricles. The third letter informs us that the pacemaker is able to be inhibited and be triggered (D = dual). The fourth letter (C) refers to its communicative or telemetry properties. It also tells us that it is multi-programmable. (A DDDMP would not possess telemetry nor shock function). The fifth letter refers to its anti-tachyarrhythmia function.

A DDDRO pacemaker, in addition to dual chamber pacing, dual chamber sensing and a dual response to sensing, would have rate adaptiveness.

An OOOPD would be a programmable (P) device with anti-tachy pacing and shock (D) capabilities. Such a device would be a programmable Automatic Implantable Cardioverter/Defibrillator without pacing. More commonly known as an AICD

A VVIPD would be a combination of a VVIP pacemaker i.e. ventricular paced/ ventricular sensed, inhibited with simple programmability and an AICD (that has dual anti-tachy pacing and shock functions). Commonly known as a *PCD* or Pacing Cardiovertor/Defibrillator.

Knowledge of the NBG code is a pre-requisite to the understanding of pacemaker function. Of seemingly less importance are the electrodes that are connected to the pacemaker and although they do not possess the same technical complexities, they are in themselves a vital component of the pacemaker system.

There are more types of electrodes available from the many manufacturers than pacemakers, consequently an electrode code is inevitably more bulky than a pacemaker code. One such seven letter code has been proposed[52] that adequately describes all present known types of electrodes, but like the pacemaker generic code, as technical advancements are made, it must continually be updated.

INDICATIONS FOR PACING

Ventricular inhibited pacemakers whether VVIP, VVIM, VVIC or VVIR are the most used of all types accounting for some 80–85 % of world implants. The remainder being A-V sequential. Almost all VVI pacemakers are programmable that will allow adjustment for pacing within the atrium (AAI).

Of the single chamber VVI types, the indications for pacing include:

❏ Complete heart block (CHB), either acquired or congenital with severe bradycardia.
❏ Second degree AV block (Mobitz type 1) if symptomatic.
❏ Second degree AV block (Mobitz type 2)
❏ Hypersensitive carotid sinus syndrome (HCSS) with dizzyness or syncope.
❏ Sinus bradycardia with symptoms.
❏ Sinus node dysfunction (sick sinus syndrome) with or without tachyarrhythmias
❏ Fascicular block with syncope in association with CHB.
❏ Overdrive pacing in patients with frequent refractory ventricular tachycardia.
❏ Atrial fibrillation with slow ventricular response.
❏ Patients in whom there is no significant haemodynamic benefit from atrial contraction.

Atrial inhibited (AAI) pacemakers are less commonly used and are likely to be indicated in sinus node dysfunction in the presence of normal A-V conduction.

Rate adaptive (VVIR) pacemakers are generally indicated for those patients with chronotropic incompetence who would be helped with an increased rate during exercise. They are becoming increasingly popular and whilst the simple single chamber muscular activity type that senses vibrations by means of a piezo-electric crystal is the most used VVIR pacemaker today it cannot increase the heart rate during exercises that do not involve the musculature surrounding the area of implantation. VVIR pacemakers do not respond well to emotional disturbances, e.g. stress or fright.

Dual chamber (DDD, DDI, DVI, VDD, DDDR). A growing number of patients are receiving dual chamber pacemakers and although there still exists much controversy amongst the experts regarding the pros and cons of VVIR versus DDD, there is a definite need of this type of pacemaker. Dual chamber pacing does relieve the symptoms that are associated with absence of A-V synchrony, such as pacemaker syndrome[53] and regurgitation during the early isovolumetric period of contraction that must impair overall cardiac efficiency.[54] It has also been shown to increase cardiac output by 24–44 % during exercise as compared with VVI pacing.[55] DDDR pacing has allowed patients with sino-atrial node dysfunction to have the benefits of rate adaptiveness with AV synchrony.

Although there have been many reported instances of inadequacies of atrial sensing, even when the pacemaker is programmed at its maximum sensitivity, and despite the real probability in many patients of the onset of atrial fibrillation, there exists no better method of pacing than one that is tracking the SA node and appropriately capturing the ventricles (chronotrophic competence). Fortunately, in the eventuality of loss of atrial sensing or the development of atrial fibrillation, most DDD pacemakers can be programmed to VVI and some more expensive models to VVIR. Certain models are able to sense an atrial tachyarrhythmia and automatically revert the mode of operation to VVI.

The VDD pacemaker utilising a single electrode is gaining some popularity. It has the pacing electrode located at its tip within the ventricle and its sensing electrode located proximally at a distance where it would be in contact with the atrial wall.

The indications for dual chamber pacemaking are:

❑ Those patients in whom sequential atrial and ventricular contractions are likely to improve their quality of life.

❑ Those patients who experience discomforting pacemaker syndrome or have experienced pacemaker syndrome with a previously implanted VVI.

❑ When VVI pacing elicits a fall in blood pressure.

❑ When retrograde conduction causes discomfort.

❑ Second or third degree heart block with otherwise healthy sinus node function.

THE PACEMAKER LEAD

To allow the pacemaker impulses to be transmitted to the heart chamber(s) an electrode lead or leads must be connected to the pacemaker. The pacemaker may be either *unipolar or bipolar*.

A unipolar pacemaker has connected to it a single conductive wire, insulated over its entire length, that transmits the impulse to its conductive distal tip; the tip being the *cathode* and the pacemaker can (the metal container) being the *anode*.

A bipolar pacemaker has two wires within the lead, each insulated from each other contained within one insulated sheath throughout its entire length. At the proximal end two in-line connectors allow the electrode to be electrically connected to the pacemaker whilst the distal portion has two exposed electrodes, one situated at the distal tip (cathode) and the other ring electrode located some 1–2 centimetres proximally (anode). In this bipolar system the pacemaker can has NO electrical connection.

The electrode connector
The proximal connectors of the electrode and likewise the pacemaker receptacle, or socket in which the electrode is inserted, are available in three common (outside diameter) sizes:

❑ The most popular 3.2 mm, is presented as *bipolar in-line* in which the two contacts are positioned one behind the other, or as *unipolar*, having a single contact. Either type may be of *Draft International Standard No. 1* configuration known as *IS-1*, having a shorter pin stem or, the less used *Voluntary Standard No. 1, VS-1* type, which conforms to a standard set by an industrial agreement.

❑ 4.75 mm which may be of the older bipolar configuration having a bifurcated proximal portion with separate contacts (uncommon), or as a unipolar, having a single contact.

❑ 5.8 mm. unipolar only with one single contact (uncommon).

❑ 6.0 mm bi-polar 'in-line' or unipolar with one single contact (obsolete).

Plastic adaptors allow smaller size connectors to be inserted into larger size sockets, but the reverse situation where a large connector is inserted into a small pacemaker socket usually necessitates the use of a bulky connector that once implanted, is likely to cause erosion through the skin, especially if the pacemaker is positioned superficially in the area of implantation of a thin patient.

Most A-V sequential pacemakers (DDD) require two separate leads in order to pace the atria and the ventricle, although few use a single lead that has an electrode situated very proximal to its distal tip, that is made to contact the atrial wall (VDD). Sometimes known as dual chamber devices they are meant to mimic the hearts physiological function, i.e. contraction of the atria prior to the ventricle. They may be unipolar or bipolar and accept electrodes accordingly. In the unipolar configuration, the distal tip of both leads would be the cathode and the pacemaker can, the anode.

NB. Passive bipolar epicardial leads are now available by some manufacturers.

Electrode lead types   Many types of pacing electrodes (sometimes known as *leads)* are available, each having special qualities generalised under two headings. They are either *epicardial,* suitable for fixation on the epicardial surface of the heart, or *endocardial* that are introduced via a superficial vein and the distal tip located within a heart chamber. Both Epi and Endocardial leads are available as unipolar or bipolar types. Insulation is usually silicon rubber or polyurethane.

Leads are subclassified according to the fixation elements of the distal tip which may be active or passive. A typical example of an epicardial active fixation electrode is the popular screw-in type electrode that has a 2¼ turn conductive metal corkscrew at the tip which is screwed into the myocardium. A less common passive fixation epicardial electrode is the 'helicoid' type that consists of a coil that horizontally lies upon the myocardial surface. It rests within a silicon platform that is sutured to the epicardial surface. It does not puncture the muscle but is applied only to the epicardial surface. Another less common active fixation is the 'stab' epicardial electrode that has a fish hook like distal tip allowing it to be inserted beneath the epicardial surface.

Endodocardial leads may also be active although most used are passive. A typical example of an endocardial active electrode is the retractable screw-in that allows the operator to screw out a small diameter corkscrew from the distal end of the electrode once a suitable site of placement has been found. Another well used active screw-in type has a soluble polyethyline glycol protective sheath that covers the screw long enough to allow correct placement within the heart chamber. On the other hand a typical passive electrode is the porous tined. The distal tip having a metallic trellis or mesh at its tip allowing in-growth of fibrin to accumulate. Plastic fins known as tines that protrude from the sides of the distal portion allow better retaining properties within the trabeculaed right ventricle. There is no invasion of the muscle.

There are a variety of electrodes available each different in design and some used only for specific purposes. Not only is the material of the tip of importance but also its ability to retain its

FIGURE 84
A pacemaker implantation in which an active unipolar epicardial electrode has been used.

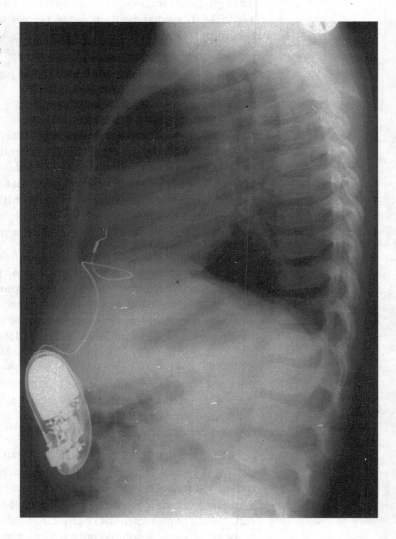

position within the heart chamber, its conductivity and insulating properties. Some of the tip materials used are:

- ❏ Platinum
- ❏ Platinum/iridium alloy
- ❏ Activated vitreous (or pyrolytic) carbon
- ❏ Elgiloy (an alloy of cobalt, nickel, chromium, molybdenum and iron.
- ❏ Stainless steel.
- ❏ Vitallium

FIGURE 85
A pacemaker implantation in which a passive bi-polar endocardial lead has been used.

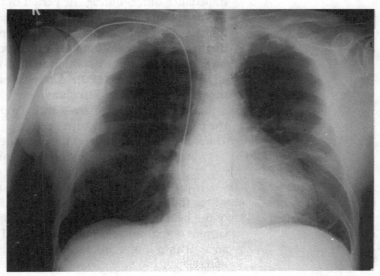

The tip design may be:

Ringed — Spherical — Porous — Cylindrical, or one of many other unique designs. Each being a compromise of the many qualities desired in an ideal electrode. As the pacing electrode transfers the energy from the pacemaker to the heart muscle, and senses any incoming signals it receives from the heart, it is important that it possesses:

1. *High current density:* Current density is the charge/second per unit surface area expressed in mA/cm^2. It is the amount of energy delivered to the myocardium and is proportional to the polarisation voltage over the surface area of the electrode tip.

2. *Low polarisation*: Polarisation is the voltage drop occurring within the interface between the electrode tip and the myocardial tissue and is caused by the concentration of charged ions at the electrode tip. It is negligible at the commencement of discharge of the impulse and increases throughout the discharge until it diffuses through the tissue as soon as the discharge is finished. It is a function of the surface area of the electrode tip.

3. *Low stimulation impedance*: The stimulation impedance, denoted by the letter Z and measured as volts/ampere or ohms, is calculated by simple Ohm's law and is the measurement of the resistance to current flow of the whole pacing system during the time of discharge of energy. This includes the electrode, the myocardial tissue and the interface. It is technically wrong to use the term 'lead impedance' as the lead (or electrode) is a fixed resistive element whilst the interface is a capacitive element.

Impedance differs during the period of impulse discharge and the period during sensing. It is of course important that the impedance of the system is not too low otherwise high current drainage will occur. Stimulation impedance should always be measured at the nominal output settings of the pacemaker, usually 5 V at 0.5 ms. i.e. if the current measured is 9.8 mA, then the impedance will be 510 ohms.

Impedance = V/I, where V is the applied output voltage of the pacemaker and I the current.

The *load* of the system = (*a*) the resistance of the electrode +
                                        (*b*) the tissue interface impedance +
                                        (*c*) polarisation impedance

where (*a*) is a pure resistive load, (*b*) the impedance at the area where the electrode is in contact with the endocardial surface of the heart and (*c*) a function of the area of the electrode tip, current amplitude and pulse duration. The higher the impedance, within limits, the less the current drain from the pacemaker.

Figure 86 shows a simple electrical circuit of the pacemaker system and the resistive elements that determine current flow and subsequent longevity. C represents the capacitive impulse discharge of a constant voltage pacemaker (Vo) having an exponential decay waveform; Re, the resistance of the pacing electrode; Zp, the impedance imposed by polarisation; and Ri the interface resistance. Io is the total current drawn within the circuit.

FIGURE 86
A simplfied circuit of a pacemaker system

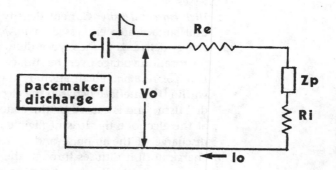

A *constant voltage* output pacemaker is one that maintains a constant voltage irrespective of applied load. There are of course limits to the amount of current that can be drawn from the pacemaker before there is a voltage drop. The majority of pacemakers are constant voltage devices that show battery depletion by one or more of the following indicators:

1. a decrease in rate discharge,
2. a decrease in the magnetic rate,
3. an increase in the pulse width, or

4. an indicatation of the degree of depletion by the use of a programmer with two-way telemetry.

ELECTROMAGNETIC INTERFERENCE (EMI)

The lead is in simple terms, a wire that transmits electrical signals
to and from the heart. The signals that originate from the pacemaker (1.0–7.5V) are much larger than those it receives from the
heart (a fraction to a few mV) and as the prime function of the
pacemaker is to:

(a) generate the voltage required to stimulate the heart, and

(b) sense incoming signals that are generated by the heart, it is
obvious that the sensing mechanism of the pacemaker must be
high enough to be able to recognise the small signals that are
transmitted from the heart chamber via the electrode(s), especially those produced within the atrium.

It is because of the high sensitivity required of the pacemaker to
recognise intrinsic electrical activity of the heart that it is inevitably
sensitive to strong external electrical sources. The electrode acts as
an antennae receiving signals that are liable to confuse the pacemaker into believing they are QRS or P complexes. The worse effect
is *inhibition* of the discharging impulses that can cause dizziness,
syncope or if prolonged, death. Much depends of course upon the
type and strength of the EMI, the proximity of the pacemaker to
the source and how dependent the patient is to pacing, i.e. whether
the patient has an underlying rhythm and how soon the heart can
establish an effective pulse. Many patients often question the possibility of their pacemakers being influenced by external electrical
interference. Most are well shielded from sources of electrical interference that the patient is likely to encounter in daily life, but some
of these may under certain circumstances, temporarily slow down
or speed up the rate. Most manufacturers have safeguarded their
pacemakers by shielding and incorporating special filters within
the circuitry to prevent their abnormal behaviour. High power
radio and ultra high frequency waves are known to affect pacemaker function and may (a) inhibit the pacemaker discharge; (b)
cause it to revert to an interference mode of action or (c) deprogram
the unit.

Strong electromagnetic radio frequency interference such as
emitted by cautery units during surgery performed in close proximity to the pacemaker, may cause severe damage to the pacemaker
amplifiers, especially to the highly sensitive atrial amplifier of an
A-V sequential pacemaker.

Fortunately the modern pacemaker is able to electronically filter most forms of EMI interferences within the radio frequency

spectrum (RF) that may be produced by a number of sources in the hospital. Clinical and medical personnel should be aware of the most common, i.e. cautery, diathermy apparatus and most electric motors that cause arcing between the commutator and brushes. It must be remembered that the *AICD* and *PCD* are equally affected by EMI and magnetic fields.

During *surgery* the pacemaker patient is especially at greater risk and the operating room staff should be familiar with the procedures to minimise any possibility of pacemaker malfunction. Generally these may be summarised:

1. Apply the indifferent cautery pad *as far away from the chest area* as possible, e.g. the buttocks or rear of the thigh. The patient with a pacemaker implanted in the area of the right pectoral fold undergoing a prostatectomy, with the indifferent pad placed under the buttocks, would be at minimal risk compared to the patient with a similar sited pacemaker undergoing a partial mastectomy of the right breast.
2. *Low output and short bursts* of cautery should be used to avoid or reduce the inhibition time should the patient be pulseless.
3. *Reprogramme an A-V sequential pacemaker to VVI* at a reduced sensitivity, or, with caution, to VOO prior to surgery. Doing so will disable the very high sensing mechanism of the atrial portion of the pacemaker. N.B. A cardiologist should be consulted prior to reprogramming.
4. *Do not cauterise over pacemaker site.*
5. Always *monitor ECG and pulse* during operation.

These rules and the effects may not apply in all circumstances as much would depend on the operation field, the site of the pacemaker and its mode of operation, and whether the patient is in continuous sinus rhythm or is *pacemaker dependent,* etc.

IMPLANTATION

The technique of endocardial implantation of a cardiac pacemaker is a relatively simple procedure and is performed at most hospitals by cardiologists or radiologists who are familiar with catheterisation of the heart. Some physicians may prefer to temporarily pace the heart prior and during implantation of a permanent device. It is well to be reminded of two conditions when a new pacemaker should never be implanted.

❑ If stored outside of the temperatures range of 0–50 °C, or
❑ if accidentally dropped onto a hard surface.

Using local anaesthesia, a cutdown is made that is large enough to accommodate the pacemaker in the selected region of the body.

The usual site for an endocardial approach is the right or, less frequently, the left infraclavicular area. The upper quadrant of the rectus sheath of the abdomen is the common site of choice for epicardial placement.

If a right sided placement is chosen a tributary of the brachiocephalic vein, or subclavian vein, is located and an appropriate electrode introduced. Under x-ray guidance the distal tip of the electrode is pushed until its tip is firmly in contact with the endocardial surface of the right ventricular apex.

After electrical threshold measurements of the electrode and the appropriate intrinsic (if any) P and/or R wave amplitudes are measured, the output parameters of the pacemaker are checked. If a unipolar pacemaker is used it may be advisable to pace the heart with the *pacing system analyser* at the output voltage of the pacemaker, i.e. 5 V to ensure that there is no diaphragmatic excitation of surrounding muscle, commonly known as *twitching*. The electrode is then inserted into the 'boot' of the pacemaker and screwed home. Once connected, the operator should give a gentle 'tug' to the electrode at its proximal end, making sure that it is firmly attached within its orifice. A silk tie is made around the boot of the pacemaker to ensure a fluid seal. A subcutaneous 'pocket' large enough to allow the pacemaker to lie flat against the chest wall is made and the pacemaker with connected electrode inserted. It is important that any extra portion of the electrode be neatly coiled without a twist and placed beneath the pacemaker during insertion. If a unipolar system is used, the pacemaker plate or 'window' (anode) should lie away from the musculature. The wound is then sutured and the operation completed.

Other methods of electrode routing may be necessary, e.g. a subclavian approach if the cephalic is too narrow to accept an electrode. A transmural approach if the patient has SVC obstruction or a mechanical prosthetic tricuspid valve. Such a description of implantation is of course over-simplified and does not take into account the operator skills and technical expertise required, especially when implanting an A-V sequential device or dealing with complications that are sometimes encountered. The reader is advised to consult recommended literature.

The measurement of threshold Once the electrode tip is within the chamber of the right ventricle and located within the apex (assuming an endocardial implant) it is important that the *stimulation threshold* be measured. This is the lowest level of electrical energy that will consistently cause capture of the heart, i.e. depolarisation of the chamber. It is measured as voltage (V) or current (mA) at the nominal pulse width of the pacemaker that is implanted, usually 0.5 ms. This test is performed to ensure that the electrode is in an electrically correct position.

Should the patient be temporarily paced, the external pacemaker should be switched off during this procedure. A decremental analyzer, commonly referred to as a pacing system analyzer (PSA) is connected to the proximal connectors of the electrode and, assuming there is 1:1 capture, the voltage is slowly reduced from 5 V (the output of most pacemakers) to zero. During which time the ECG is continually monitored to notice when capture ceases, i.e. when the pacemaker impulse or spike is NOT followed by a QRS complex. That point is the *pacing threshold*. This lowest voltage should be noted together with the pulse width at which measurement was taken.

It is also important to measure and note the current value, at the point of threshold, which is usually a little higher than the voltage figure.

A typical threshold of an endocardial ventricular electrode might be 0.5V and 0.7mA at 0.5ms duration, giving a resistance of 714 ohms (R=V/I). The output of the analyser should immediately be returned to a safe voltage after this is determined.

REMEMBER

The technologist should be aware of the possible consequences of performing this test on patients who do not have an adequate escape rhythm or equally important, are likely to develop tachyarrhythmias during asystolic periods. Should the patient, for example, be in sinus rhythm at a high rate, thresholds may still be determined by *overdriving* the sinus rhythm at a paced rate of ±10 % higher than his intrinsic rate.

The acceptable threshold values for endocardial stimulation are usually less than 1 volt and often around 0.5 V. Epicardial threshold values are often higher and 1.5 V may be acceptable.

Next, the sensing threshold should be measured. This can only be attained when intrinsic R waves are present. It may be calculated by the analyser which will give the amplitude of the QRS complex as measured at the distal tip of the implanted electrode, OR the technologist may wish to record the height of the intra-ventricular electrogram more accurately by attaching the proximal connector of the electrode to the Wilson V electrocardiograph lead terminal. Provided the ECG channel is correctly calibrated, i.e. 1mV=1cm, the height in mVolts can be measured. It should be well in excess of the maximal sensitivity of the pacemaker. Ventricular amplitudes may vary between 1 and 25 mV.

The electrode is then connected to the pacemaker.

The strength duration curve In order to conserve energy from the pacemaker it may, under certain circumstances, be advantageous to select or program the

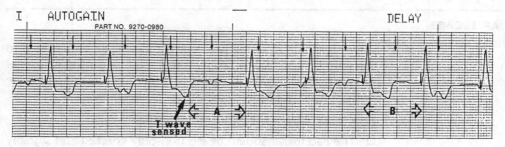

FIGURE 87

Inhibition of the VVIM pacemaker due to oversensing. The sensitivity of the generator has been programmed too high, i.e. it senses the unwanted T wave which is of much lower amplitude than its QRS.

pacemaker to various amplitudes and pulse widths. This test, often performed some six weeks after implantation informs the physician of the stable settings at which the pacemaker can safely capture the heart. It is a continuous plot of impulse voltage (or current) to progressive impulse duration lengths. The 'rheobase' is the minimum point of amplitude plotted against an infinitely long duration. The 'chronaxie pulse duration time' is twice the value of the rheobase.

FIGURE 88
The Strength Duration
Curve

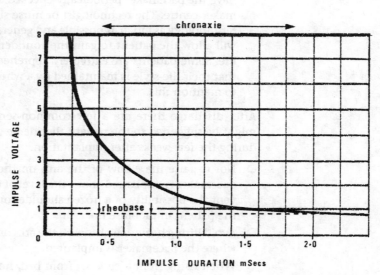

AFTERCARE

After implantation of the pacemaker, and the patient returned to the ward, care should be taken by all attending clinical personnel to avoid supporting or lifting the patient under the armpit on the side of the body where the pacemaker is implanted.

Prior to discharge of the patient from hospital:

❑ The pacemaker should be electronically checked and suitably programmed

❑ An ECG with rhythm strip recorded

❑ Two chest x-rays of high penetration, one in the AP and the other in the lateral view, should be taken as controls for future use

❑ The patient should be informed of the reasons WHY a pacemaker has been implanted and WHY it is important that he or she check the pulse at regular intervals. HOW, in simple language, it should behave and if not, WHAT symptoms will he or she experience, and WHEN the battery depletes HOW he or she will recognise it. It should be stressed HOW important it is to have the pacemaker periodically checked at a recognised pacemaker centre. The technologist or nurse should avoid medical terminology as much as possible and generate an assurance that will allow the patient to gain the confidence to lead a normal life. Some patients are extremely apprehensive at the thought that their life-style is maintained by a wire, although reluctant to mention this.

After discharge there are a few common-sense precautions that might be suggested to the patient that he be requested to observe during the few weeks after implantation:

❑ Not to raise the elbow of the arm on the side on which the pacemaker is implanted above the level of the shoulder. To prevent the possibility of a frozen shoulder on no account should the patient immobilise the arm.

❑ Avoid lifting heavy weights with the arm on the side of his body where the pacemaker is implanted.

❑ When rising from a chair or from bed, not to use this arm to assist his rising.

The patient is asked to observe these precautions for two special reasons. Firstly, by not rotating the arm or raising it above the shoulder after implantation, it is unlikely that the electrode tip located within the heart, will become dislodged. Electrode dislodgement is an uncommon complication that is usually experienced within the first few weeks after its implantation. Fibrous growth, caused by rejection of the foreign substance soon attaches it to the endocardial tissue (figure 89).

Secondly, by not lifting heavy weights or supporting his body with the arm, contraction of the pectoralis major is avoided, allowing the chest wound to heal more readily. Once the wound has healed and there are no complications (sepsis, oozing) the patient may use the arm naturally.

❑ Not to touch the implantation area with fingers, nor to later fiddle with the pacemaker. Fingers are generally dirty and are likely to contaminate the raw wound.

❑ The patient is advised to keep a regular check on his pulse. It is preferred that this be done before getting out of bed (when the pacemaker is more likely to be functioning in the absence of any intrinsic rhythm higher than the preprogrammed pacemaker rate). It should be felt at the wrist and counted over a period of one minute, using the second hand of a watch. He should be informed of the function of his particular pacemaker and what to do and whom to contact should he experience any dizzyness or syncope.

❑ It is of course important that the patient be aware of the possible, although unlikely, event of electromagnetic interference (EMI) causing his pacemaker to malfunction.

Let us first list the potential sources of electrical interference that should not affect the pacemaker:

Household appliances	*Air conditioners *Blender/food processing machine/mixers *Can openers *Washing machines/clothes driers *Dish washers *Electric bread knives Electric heaters *Sewing machines Television/stereo/remote controls Radio receivers/CD players
Power tools	*Band saws *Drill presses *Electric generators *Lathes *Milling machines *Polishers *Sand blasters *Sanders *Surface grinders

Helium arc welding equipment
*Hedge trimmers
*Lawn mowers

External sources   *Garage door opening devices
*Power generating plant
TV/radio stations
Theft protection devices (as found in retail stores and libraries).

Note: The appliances mentioned above marked with an asterisk (*) are operated by electric motors which do emit low power radio frequencies. Although they are highly unlikely to affect the pacemaker it is necessary to advise the patient not to allow the pacemaker to be within 20 cm of any motor.

The following advice may be also considered:

A home *microwave oven* may be used. It is highly unlikely to affect the pacemaker unless the door seals are worn and microwaves be radiated towards the pacemaker, which event may change the programmed parameters. As an precaution the patient may be advised to retreat from the oven once it is switched on.

High powered electrical equipment such as arc welders and plasma cutters should be used with caution. If the occupation of the patient is dependent on the use of such equipment it would be advisable to contact the pacemaker manufacturer. Much depends on the type of pacemaker, its site within the body and how it is programmed.

Care should be taken when using an *electric hand drill*. It may be unwise to hold it in close proximity to the pacemaker site. i.e. less than 20 cm.

An *electric razor* may also be safely used but it should not be held close to the area of the implant site when switched on.

The use of an *electric blanket* is permissible although it is advised to be used only for warming the bed prior to entering.

A *cellular telephone* may affect the pacemaker. It should not be carried close to the pacemaker or electrodes, and should be at least 20 cm from the pacemaker when used.

Driving a motor car. The ignition system of a car *will not* affect the pacemaker function whilst driving although it is advised that the patient does not lean over the open bonnet (hood) of the engine while it is turning especially if the pacemaker is located in the pectoral region. It is recommended that a seat belt be worn at all times. A tight belt that would cause chafing over the pacemaker site is not advised. Traffic authorities will usually only give exemption from wearing a seat belt on the advice of a medical specialist.

Radar equipment used by traffic police will not normally affect the operation of the pacemaker but the patient is advised not to approach the close proximity of broadcasting *antennae,* e.g. high powered radio and television transmitters, and amateur or CB radio transmitting equipment.

Air travel. Travel on all commercial aircraft is permitted. Such travel will not affect the pacemaker.

Gun or metal detector devices such as those commonly found at airport terminals will not adversely affect the operation of the pacemaker. However it will be detected by the metal detector and for the patient's own convenience he or she should inform the airport officials prior to entering the screen. Proof may be required by airport security, e.g. Medic-alert bracelet, hospital document, etc.

Medical treatment Should the patient require medical treatment that uses *diathermy* equipment he must inform the doctor that he has an implanted cardiac pacemaker. The interference generated from this type of equipment may seriously harm the pacemaker. *radiofrequency ablation* techniques when an *electrosurgical unit* or an *ablator* is used would not be carried out without the knowledge of a cardiologist.

Should the patient need to undergo *surgery* of any kind it is important that the surgeon be informed that he has an implanted pacemaker.

High energy ionizing radiation sources such as cobalt-60 or those produced by a linear accelerator (used for cancer treatment) may seriously affect the CMOS circuitry of the pacemaker. Gamma rays should never be directed at the pacemaker. It is advised, however, to shield the pacemaker site with *x*-ray apron material.

Care should be taken when *mega voltage radiation* of any form is used. This includes *deep x*-ray therapy (DXT). The patient should be ECG monitored and on no account should radiation be directed near to the pacemaker or electrode(s) sites.

Should the patient require *magnetic resonance imaging (MRI),* constant monitoring during the evaluation must be carried out. This procedure has been shown to cause movement of the pacemaker within the subcutaneous pocket, and/or to deprogram the device or cause temporary asynchonous pacing.

Should the patient have an *automatic implantable cardioverter/ defibrillator(AICD)* or *PCD,* MRI will probably deactivate the unit, causing the patient to lose arrhythmia or defibrillation protection. It is also important that (*a*) bi-polar pacing be used when an AICD is implanted and (*b*) it is not advisable to use a pacemaker that will revert to unipolar pacing during the presence of electrical interference of any kind.

Transcutaneous electric nerve stimulators (TENS) are generally contra-indicated. If used it is important that (*a*) the electrodes be placed as close to each other and as far from the pacemaker system as possible and (*b*) the output be monitored and adjusted to cause no pacemaker malfunction prior to the patient leaving the hospital/clinic/rooms.

Should *cardioversion/defibrillation* be necessary it is important to observe the usual precautions (see chapter defibrillation).

X-rays will not affect the pacemaker.

A *hearing aid* will not affect the pacemaker.

Lithotripsy should never be applied over or near to the implanted pacemaker.

Dental treatment   Many pacemaker patients enquire whether dental equipment can interfere with the function of cardiac pacemakers and generally it is not likely to occur. The use of electric burr drives and ultrasound scaling devices do not interfere with pacemaker function. However high frequency surgical devices and electric pulp function testers may affect the pacemaker. Any instruments and machines that operate with high frequency electric or magnetic fields should not be located in close proximity to the pacemaker.

> It must be noted, however, that there are many important factors that determine whether or not electromagnetic interference is likely to affect pacemaker function.
>
> ❑ The type of pacemaker implanted,
> ❑ Its preprogrammed parameter levels (especially sensitivity),
> ❑ The site of the pacemaker and the polarity and configuration of the electrodes and,
>   The power and frequency of the radiating source.

Follow-up   After routine removal of sutures and re-application of wound dressing, the patient should return to the clinic within a period of a few weeks for assessment of his physical condition, to measure the threshold and if necessary, further reprogramming of his pacemaker. NB. Extension of pacemaker longevity may be attained by either decreasing the pulse width or decreasing the voltage. *Remember, decreasing the pulse width will proportionally decrease the delivered energy, i.e energy is proportional to pulse width. Decreasing the output voltage will decrease the energy four times, i.e. energy delivered is directly proportional to the square of the amplitude.*

Pacing thresholds may be measured with the use of a handheld programmer that will allow the operator to change programmable functions by placing the device over the site of the implanted pacemaker. Many programmers have automatic threshold capabilities allowing a stepwise decrease of the voltage output. Monitoring will show the point of non-capture and will allow resumption of nominal pacing as soon as the programmer is removed from the vicinity

FIGURE 89

Autopsy photograph showing the encasement of an electrode within fibrotic tissue some years after implantation. Such an electrode would have been extremely difficult to remove by mechanical means.

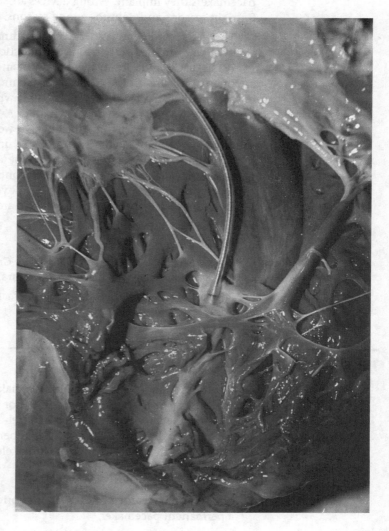

of the pacemaker. Some need the operator to manually reset the nominal parameters by pressing a soft switch on the fascia of the instrument. It is not advised to perform threshold measurements alone, especially if the patient is dependent upon the pacemaker. Always work with an assistant nearby and have CPR equipment at hand, which should include a transcutaneous pacemaker.

The technology associated with cardiac pacing is complex and at times confusing. It does not always provide the maximum comfort to the patient. Doctors themselves who are intimately involved with the art are often unable to understand the operation of many pacemakers they implant. Wrong devices are sometimes implanted for right reasons and right for wrong reasons.

The electrocardiograms are often a nightmare to interpret especially when combined with intrinsic conduction aberrations. Those of DVI, DDDCP, and certain types of VVIR and DDDR pacemakers are often confusing to the clinician or technologist. The addition of such parameters as Vario function, safety windows, fallback, rate smoothing, PVARP extension, dynamic A-V delay, anti-tachy response with mode switching etc, make it worse. Added to this is the inability of manufacturers to supply a universal programmer that will allow the operator to programme any of the scores of pacemakers available. There is still much controversy amongst the experts regarding the pros and cons of VVIR versus DDD pacing. It has been suggested that VVIR pacemakers are rarely scientifically programmed.[56]

Further reading

❑ Levine PA & Mace RC. *Pacing Therapy. A Guide to Cardiac Pacing for Optimum Haemodynamic Benefit.* Futura. New York. 1983.

❑ Furman S, Hayes DL & Holmes DR. *A Practice of Cardiac Pacing.* Futura. New York. 1986.

THE EXTERNAL PACEMAKER

Unlike the permanent implantable pacemaker, the *temporary* or *external pacemaker* is an electronic stimulator powered by disposable alkaline, mercury or re-chargeable nickel-cadmium batteries. It is bulky, uses hybrid circuitry and like its permanent counterpart may be used with endocardial or epicardial electrodes.

It is used specifically for the treatment of:

❑ Transient bradycardias or arrhythmias prior to the insertion of a permanent pacemaker,

❑ Patients with acute myocardial infarction who are likely to present with complete heart block or any one of many conduction disturbances,

❑ Patients who have bradycardia associated with drug toxicity or low output states.

❑ Patients who develop complete heart block during cardiac surgery.

❑ Refractory tachycardias when suppression is often obtained by electrical overdriving, i.e. at a rate higher than the arrhythmia.

❑ It may also be used as a temporary relief of carotid sinus syndrome.

There are many types of electrodes available for an *endocardial* approach:

❑ The *floating* electrode is a very thin and pliable insulated wire that is allowed to float upstream to the right ventricular apex.

❑ The *balloon* electrode is a flow-directed type that has a balloon located at its distal tip. After introduction into a superficial vein the electrode is gently pushed so that the balloon is positioned within the superior vena cava. The balloon is then inflated and encouraged to float into the right atrium, through the tricuspid valve until the exposed conductive tip rests in the right ventricular apex in contact with the endocardial surface.

❑ The *guided* is the most commonly used of temporary electrodes. It is more stiff than most and not as pliable as its permanent counterpart. It is made of a nylon weave inner core surrounded by a gum elastic cover which allows good torque transference during its insertion under x-ray guidance.

Most external endocardial pacing electrodes are bipolar that have their distal tip electrodes either 1 cm (NBIH) or 1 inch (USCI Goetz) apart and are usually introduced into the ante-cubital vein of the right arm. The pacemaker is strapped to the upper or lower portion of the patients arm or, using an extension connecting cable, to a convenient part of the bedrail. At the proximal end of the electrode(s) are two pin connectors that allow the electrode to be fixed to the pacemaker.

Epicardial attachment of the electrodes may be performed by a sub-ziphoid approach, thoracotomy, sternotomy, or may be attached directly to the anterior right ventricular wall at the time of cardiac surgery. The system may be unipolar or bipolar depending upon the approach and ease of electrode placement. Should a unipolar system be used, perhaps because of limited space of heart on which to apply more than one electrode, the active electrode is connected to the negative terminal of the pacemaker and a second indifferent needle electrode inserted sub- cutaneously, is connected to the positive terminal of the pacemaker.

Functionally, the temporary pacemaker behaves exactly like the programmable permanent type. Most are VVI's although some manufacturers do supply DDD or DVI versions which require two electrodes to be placed in the heart, one in the right atrium and the other within the ventricle. A common atrial electrode is the 'J' design. Because of its J shaped tip, is easily positioned in the appendage of the right atrium. Combined atrial and ventricular pacing may be obtained with the use of a single catheter having six electrodes, two of these four are positioned at the tip and the other four spaced to rest against the right lateral endocardial surface of the right atrium.

FIGURE 90
Three different types of external battery operated temporary pacemakers. (L-R) Cordis VVI with x5 rate facility, Medtronic VVI and Biotronic DDD. All types accomodate 2mm pin connectors.

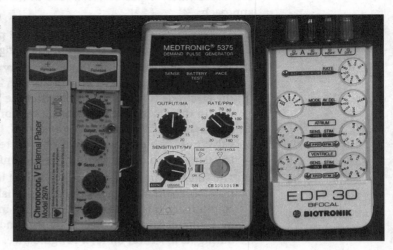

FIGURE 90
Three different types of external battery operated temporary pacemakers. (L-R) Cordis VVI with x5 rate facility, Medtronic VVI and Biotronic DDD. All types accomodate 2mm pin connectors.

The *controls* of the temporary VVI pacemaker are all manually operated and located on the fascia. They include:

❑ The on/off switch is usually a push button with a metal slide. The button is therefore always in the off position unless the metal slide covers the button to maintain the on position.

❑ The rate control adjusts the rate of the discharge of the impulses and may be varied according to the needs of the patient. The usual limits are 30–150 although it is possible on selected types to increase the rate by multiples of 3.

❑ The pulse width is usually preset on most types at approximately 1.7 ms but may be variable between 0.1 and 2.0 ms.

❑ The output control is calibrated in milliamperes or volts and is used to adopt a suitable rating above threshold. This is determined in the same manner as for permanent lead implantation, i.e. the output is turned its maximum position, then gradually decreased until capture ceases, i.e. the point when the pacemaker impulse or spike is not succeeded by a QRS complex. The output should then be increased to approximately 2–2½ times the threshold level. It is important that the patient be adequately ECG monitored during this test. Because of the likely increase in threshold values during the acute period after implantation, especially when pacing via epicardial electrodes, it is recommended that threshold measurements be taken every 12 hours.

❑ The sensitivity control is calibrated in millivolts. It is a measurement of the response of the pacemaker to intrinsic conduction. For example, a sensitivity set at 1 mV means that the pacemaker will sense all signals it receives of amplitude greater than 1 mV, which will cause it to inhibit. To any signal of lesser amplitude than 1 mV, it cannot inhibit. Let us look at the intracardiac QRS pattern. Depending upon the location of the electrode tip and, of course, many other factors such as the axis and possible infarction sites, etc, the QRS complex may, for example be over 4 mV in amplitude as seen in relation to the bipolar electrode located within the right ventricular apex. The T wave may likewise be 2 mV high. Should the sensitivity of the pacemaker be adjusted to 1mV in this instance, it would not only sense the QRS but also the T wave. This would cause prolonged extension of inhibition of the pacemaker resulting in a reduction in the rate. If on the other hand the sensitivity were to be increased to 3 mV, the T wave would not be recognised. Should the sensitivity of the pacemaker be set too high, e.g., 10 mV, then neither would be sensed and any intrinsic rhythm would not be recognised. This would cause pacemaker impulses to be superimposed on any rhythm that might be generated by the heart — an unsafe situation.

Sensitivity is an important control and should not be used indiscriminately. It is poor technology to assume that maximum sensitivity is required and to rotate the control to the most sensitive position if the patient has an intrinsic rhythm. Many patients once paced become 'addicted' to pacing and show no signs of any underlying rhythm. Sensitivity is of lesser importance to such patients and may be turned to maximum. *Note:* This control is turned clockwise for maximum sensitivity. i.e. 1 mV is a higher sensitivity than 10 mV.

❏ Few external pacemakers have a hysteresis control allowing the patients intrinsic rate to decrease to a value less than the programmed rate at which the pacemaker is set. Imagine a patient who has a sinus rhythm at a rate of 75 and has bradycardic episodes that decrease his rate to 50, and his external pacemaker is set at 70. Under normal circumstances whenever his rate falls below 70 the pacemaker would operate at 70 bpm. With the hystersis control set 60 bpm, the pacemaker would not operate until the sinus rate reached 60. At that point the pacemaker would deliver impulses at the preset rate of 70 bpm. Some patients benefit from the natural sinus rhythm at a lower rate than the artificial rhythm of pacing. The interval of 1000 ms (60 bpm) would be the hysteresis escape interval (HEI) and is that interval when the pacemaker delivers its first stimulus of its shorter automatic rate of 70. This form of pacing is not commonly used but is beneficial in selected patients.

6 *Defibrillation, Cardioversion and Ablation*

INTRODUCTION

Defibrillation is the technique of terminating fibrillation of either the atria or ventricles or both, by means of a high energy electric DC shock that is delivered through the heart. Fibrillation of the ventricles is a fatal arrhythmia that is often associated with coronary artery disease, acute myocardial infarction or with acute ectopic disturbances of cardiac rhythm. It may also be induced by drugs, electric shock, electrolytic disturbances and the many conditions that affect myocardial metabolism.

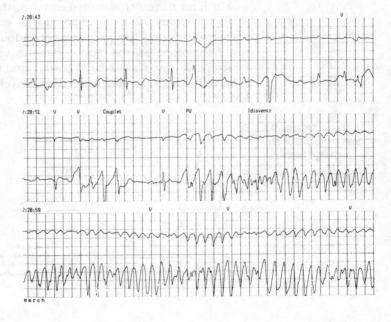

FIGURE 91
The onset of ventricular fibrillation (Torsade de Pointes) recorded from a 24 h Holter telemetry recorder

The defibrillator is the electrical instrument that is used to deliver the high energy *DC shock* which may be discharged *internally* i.e. directly across the organ via concave paddles, (with effective CPR, it is rarely necessary to internally defibrillate except when the chest is opened during cardiothoracic surgery) or *externally* i.e. indirectly via flat paddles positioned on the chest wall.

FIGURE 92
The simplified circuit of the DC defibrillator. C represents the high voltage capacitor that is charged from the transformer. When switched to the patient, the capacitor discharges through the impedence Z created by the patient.

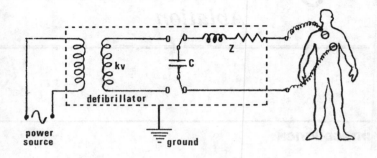

The instrument may be powered from an AC power supply or an internal battery source. In either situation the power is used to provide a direct current (DC) voltage to energise, or charge, a high voltage capacitor. The output of the defibrillator is therefore not an absolute D.C. signal but one resembling the discharge pattern of an electrical capacitor.

Much controversy has existed regarding the shape and duration of the waveform and also the amount of voltage that should be discharged. During the past decades various shaped waveforms have been proposed, the most commonly used being the underdamped half wave sinusoidal of Lown,[57] and the critically damped pulse with a high rise time and comparatively slow decay time of Edmark.[58]

FIGURE 93
Various defibrillator discharge patterns.

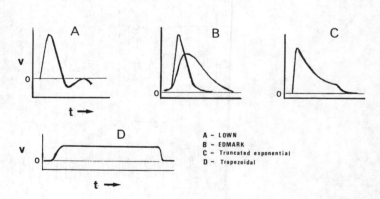

Once the paddles are positioned on the chest wall discharge is given by simultaneous depression of a button on each of two paddles. The effect of such a defibrillatory shock causes all the fibres of cardiac mus. le to become refractory and so prevent continuation of the fatal arrhythmia. Once quiescence of the cardiac muscle is established, the normal pacemaker of the heart usually responds and resumes a bradycardic rhythm .

FIGURE 94
Sinus bradycardia after delivery of a 300 joule shock.

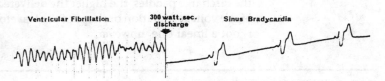

The basic instrument consists of: (*a*) an on/off switch, (*b*) an output regulator, which may be in the form of a rotating knob or push button switch, (*c*) an analogue or digital meter that will indicate the amount of energy stored by the capacitor as *joules or watt-seconds,* (both units being equivalent) and (*d*) an input paddle socket that will permit connection of the external or internal paddles to the instrument.

Each of the two paddles consists of a metal plate, which must contact the patient's chest, supported by a convenient insulated handle with buttons located on each for discharge of the shock and, on some models a switch for charging of the unit.

Ohm's law   A knowledge of Ohm's law is necessary to understand the fundamentals of the defibrillator for it is this law that governs the electrical energy that will effect defibrillation. Most defibrillators operate at output levels below 3 500 V at impulse durations from 2–15 ms.

Let us assume that a defibrillator has a maximum output voltage of 3 500 V when adjusted to an energy level of 360 joules. Let us also assume after the application of a suitable conductive gel the impedance of the chest between the applied paddles is 100 ohms, then the current can be readily calculated by Ohm's law:

$$I \text{ (current)} = \frac{3500}{100} = 35 \text{ amperes} \qquad \left(I = \frac{V}{R} \right)$$

The amount of power dissipated across the chest would be:

$$V \times I \quad \text{i.e. } 3500 \times 35 = 122\,500 \text{ W}$$

Assuming the duration of the discharged pulse to be 3.0 ms, then the energy produced would be watts × time or

$$122\,500 \times 0.003 = 367 \text{ joules}$$

Compared to the power of a household lamp (100 W) it is not difficult to realise that the defibrillator is a potentially hazardous instrument that should only be used by experienced health care personnel. The output of most DC defibrillators when set to maximum is in the order of 150 000 W of electrical power discharging some 30 amperes of electrical current across the patient's chest. Ohm's law therefore rules that the lower the impedance between the discharge paddles, the higher the delivered current, irrespective of the voltage, duration or shape of the waveform. This relationship is not a linear one, however.

DEFIBRILLATION TECHNIQUE

Defibrillation of the heart is often used to revert life-threatening arrhythmias, the most common being ventricular fibrillation (VF). Fibrillation may affect (a) the heart as a whole i.e. the involvement of both atria and ventricles (common after electrocution); (b) only the ventricles when, provided that cardiac perfusion is effectively maintained by CPR, the atria may continue to depolarise or (c) only the atria (atrial fibrillation, AF), such as may occur in the presence of severe atrial hypertrophy.

The electrocardiograph pattern of VF is characterised by irregular, completely unco-ordinated electrical artefacts that vary in time and amplitude. As time progresses, the frequency and amplitude of the aberrant waveform decreases, when the pattern is termed *agonal*. All clinical personnel should be familiar with the electrocardiographic pattern that this arrhythmia produces.

Once this fatal arrhythmia is established it is important that defibrillation be immediately effected. The sooner it is carried out the more likely it will be effective. The defibrillator should be switched on and an adequate power setting (see below) adjusted by means of the power output control. Approximately 5 cm. of a suitable defibrillator conductive paste should be squeezed from the tube on each of the defibrillator paddles which should then be positioned with firm pressure on the correct areas of the chest.

Electrode application Distribution of the gel over the entire area of the metal portion of the paddles is essential prior to their application to the chest wall. This may be attained by placing the plates together and rotating them in a circular motion, or to apply the gelled electrodes to the chest wall and then rotate them. Either way, it is *important* to break down the electrical resistance that the skin offers to avoid possible burns.

NOTE | *Do not use gels or pastes that are not recommended for defibrillation,* such as Ultrasound gel, some ECG creams, KY jelly. Most of these gels or pastes do not have sufficient conductivity and may cause severe erythema.

Any dry areas between the electrode and the patient is likely to cause redness or burning of the skin. Too much paste or gel applied to the electrodes on the other hand may spill over the electrode as it is applied to the chest wall and possibly cause a short circuit of each of the electrodes.

Should this occur it is likely to produce arcing and a spark to be seen to dissipate the current across the chest of the patient between the two electrodes. Apart from startling the operator, the shock will often cause ineffective defibrillation of the heart and may damage the defibrillator and/or injure the patient.

CAUTION

Should it be necessary after repeated shocks, to re-apply paste to the electrode surfaces, it is *important* that the areas between the electrode sites be dried with a towel to avoid the possibility of a short-circuit of the high voltage shock.

As soon as the defibrillator paddles are in position and a pressure of approximately 10 kgm applied, the operator should inform everyone to stand clear and not to touch the patient's body nor any metallic portion of the bed whilst defibrillation is undertaken. During the discharge of such high energy there exists a large electromagnetic field within the confines of the thoracic cage that may leak to the bed chassis. (An electric shock may be felt if touched). The operator then depresses the two buttons located on each of the paddles simultaneously causing the defibrillatory shock to be discharged to the patient.

Positioning the paddles The correct placement of the paddles is usually accepted as:

1. slightly to the right of the upper portion of the sternum — the manubrium, and

2. at the region of the apex of the heart.

It is preferable that these areas be chosen although defibrillation is often successful when administering the shock at any opposite sites across the chest wall. It is however, important that the defibrillator paddles should not be positioned in close proximity to each other.

At the time of defibrillation it is common for the thorax to rise due to the depolarisation of thoracic musculature. Once the shock has been delivered the ECG monitor should be checked to ensure that defibrillation has been successful. Do not remove the paddles from the chest wall if the defib monitor allows the ECG to be recorded via the paddles.

FIGURE 95

The correct paddle positions

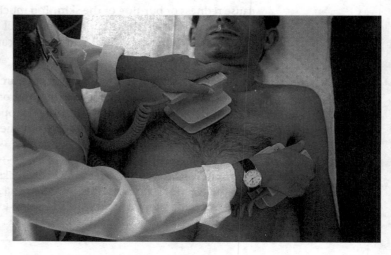

What is the correct amount of energy to use?

As a general rule the smaller the patient's size the less power is necessary to effect defibrillation. Thus for a child of approx. 5 years, no more than 50 joules is usually necessary, whereas an adult may require between 100 and 360 joules.

The American Heart Association has recommended that a delivered energy of 3.5–6.0 joules/kg of body weight should be used. It should be remembered however, that the effectiveness of defibrillation may depend upon many factors apart from body weight and thoracic size, e.g. the state of perfusion of the coronary vessels, myocardial tone, adequate oxygen exchange, etc.

From an electrical point of view, it is important to realise that it is the delivered current in amperes and not the energy in watt-seconds that effects defibrillation. The resistance, or more correctly the impedance between the two electrode paddles determines how much current is discharged and is mainly related to the resistance of the skin. Size of the electrodes also has a bearing; the smaller the electrodes the higher the resistance, thus within limits the larger the electrode the better success with defibrillation.

Another important point is the presence or absence of previous shocks. The first shock always encounters the highest skin resistance that will drop progressively with each successive shock. A defibrillator that delivers marginal current for defibrillation on the first shock is frequently effective on the second or third. It is therefore often unnecessary to increase the power output of the defibrillator when a second or third shock is given. In emergency situations it is recommended that an initial shock to an average size adult should be in the order of 200 to 250 joules. If unsuccessful the second shock should be given at the same output. The third shock may be increased by 50 joules and thereafter the maximum output of the defibrillator should be used.

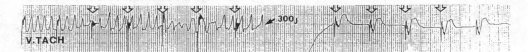

FIGURE 96

Cardioversion of a ventricular tachycardia of a patient who has an implanted pacemaker. The arrows show the discharge impulses before and after the DC shock, when subsequent pacing resumes.

SYNCHRONISED CARDIOVERSION

During ventricular fibrillation the ECG appears irregular and erratic and there are no identifiable P, Q, R, S, or T waves. In the absence of T waves the defibrillatory shock can therefore be delivered at random at any portion of the 'non-existent' cardiac cycle. However, arrhythmias other than VF, (ventricular tachycardia, flutter, atrial fibrillation, flutter) there are identifiable ventricular wave forms and a *vulnerable period* exists during the cardiac cycle. In order to avoid discharging an impulse during this period it is necessary to synchronise or trigger the discharge to occur at a time that is *not* coincident with the vulnerable period.

FIGURE 97
The vunerable zones of the cardiac cycle when mechanical or electrical stimulation may precipitate arrhythmias

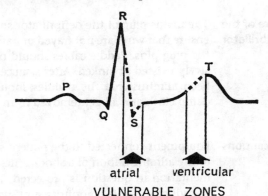

VULNERABLE ZONES

When using the defibrillator as a cardioverter it is important that the patient's electrocardiogram be monitored and the defibrillator be synchronised to sense the R wave and to immediately discharge an impulse, i.e. during depolarisation of the ventricular myocardium. As the buttons of the paddles are depressed the defibrillator hesitates until it senses the next R wave of the ECG before discharging the shock, thereby avoiding discharge during the vulnerable period.

Should the defibrillator not possess a cardioversion facility, the standard defibrillation procedure may be used. The probability of an arrhythmia reverting to ventricular fibrillation after the administration of a shock is minimal. Factors such as the patients susceptibility, heart rate and metabolic circumstances greatly influence the risk. However, the operator should be ready to immediately give a second shock should it be necessary.

Testing the defibrillator

The *only method* by which the output of a DC defibrillator may be checked is with the use of a defibrillator tester. This instrument will register the amount of energy produced by the defibrillatory discharge either as stored or delivered energy. Most defibrillators have built-in testers allowing the discharge to be dissipated across a 50 ohm load. Should your defibrillator not have such an attachment it should be regularly checked with a commercially available external tester.

On no account should a defibrillator be tested by discharging the shock whilst shorting the paddles together or holding them apart. This means of checking does not prove to the operator that the discharge shock is being transmitted to the paddles and may be harmful to the machine.

Care of the defibrillator

The mains plug of the defibrillator should be regularly checked to ensure that wires are not frayed or have become disconnected from the plug pins. Paddle cables should never be allowed to be excessively twisted or kinked. After a successful defibrillatory shock has been administered the paddles should be wiped with a slightly damp cloth and all gel removed from their surfaces.

Safety precautions

Equipment connected to the patient should be disconnected prior to the administration of a shock unless it is known that the instrumentation in question is protected. This includes some electrical transducers, cardiac monitors, etc. Should the monitor not be protected against the shock or should the ECG drift excessively during the administration of a shock it may be necessary to remove the patient cable from the monitor and reinsert it immediately after shock delivery.

External heating devices such as electric blankets should be switched off.

Do not use a defibrillator in close proximity to an oxygen source or any flammable mixture. This includes flammable anaesthetics.

Other considerations

❑ *Implanted cardiac pacemakers:*
When defibrillating a patient who has an implanted cardiac pacemaker located in the right pectoral region and an electrode within the right ventricular apex it is preferable that the defibrillatory shock be administered at right angles to the electrical axis of the pacemaker-electrode system. i.e. one defibrillatory paddle be positioned to the left of the upper portion of the sternum and the other below the right breast (V4R). Discharge in this direction i.e. at right angles, will reduce the risk of possible trauma to the endocardial interface caused by inductive charges generated along the axis of the pacemaker electrode.
Never position a defibrillator paddle over the site of an implanted pacemaker.

❑ *External pacemakers:*
The same procedure should be adopted as for an implanted unit, however it is advised to disconnect the pacer electrodes before delivery of the shock to avoid possible damage to the pacemaker.

❑ *Flow directed catheters:*
These and other intracardiac catheters should, if possible, be withdrawn from the ventricular chamber before defibrillation.

❑ *Bandaging:*
Extensive thoracic bandaging may present a problem of paddle placement. Should it not be possible to remove bandaging, any flat area of the torso may be used provided the shock is delivered through the thorax. Paddles should not be positioned close together.

❑ *ECG electrodes*:
Never position paddles over monitoring electrodes.

THE IMPLANTED DEFIBRILLATOR

Much recent progress has been made during the past years in the development of the automatic implantable cardioverter defibrillator, known as the *AICD*. Not only does this device detect tachyarrhythmias and ventricular fibrillation, but also has the ability to correct these rhythms and when necessary to pace any bradycardic situation. Referred to as a PCD, its NBG code is VVICD. It is a VVI pacemaker with both communicative and multiprogrammable properties (C).

These devices are able to deliver an adequate shock (34 joules) directly to the heart via endocardial or epicardial pad electrodes or a combination of both types. It is an antitachy detector that will deliver a series of preprogrammed impulses (P) and deliver a shock

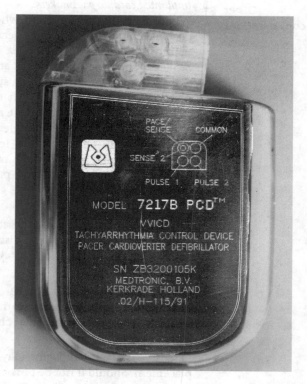

whenever ventricular fibrillation occurs (S). The fifth letter combin-
ing P and S is (D).

Because of the comparatively huge amount of energy required
to defibrillate the heart, they contain a proportionally large battery
pack and have a mass of almost 150 grams and a volume of round
80 ccs. They are implanted in the rectus sheath of the abdomen in
a similar manner as an epicardial pacemaker.

ABLATION OF THE A-V NODE BY DC SHOCK

The effect of delivery of an electric shock to the AV node was accidentally discovered by Vedel et al in 1979 during a routine electrophysiology study.[59] For almost a decade the technique of destroying
the atrio-ventricular node by means of shock administration via a
transvenous cardiac catheter has been in use and had proven to be
effective treatment (with a reported 85 % success) for supra-ventricular tachyarrhythmias that do not respond well to either pacing
or drug therapy.

Known as *DC ablation,* this *fulguration* technique involves the
introduction of a conductive pacing electrode into the right ventri-

cle where its distal portion is positioned against the septum in the region of the His bundle. Once positioned and a favourable His bundle electrogram recorded from one or more of the distal electrodes, a synchronised DC shock is administered between a chosen active electrode and a large indifferent metal electrode that is located under the left scapula. The His electrogram usually chosen is one with the a largest deflection and the longest H-V interval.

Unfortunately DC shock discharged to the heart from a standard defibrillator is not without the risk of extensive damage to the septal structure, believed to be caused by the extreme pressure changes that occur during delivery of such high electrical energy.[60] Risk is especially high when shock is delivered within the coronary sinus.[61]

Other risks include: emboli, the creation of an arrhythmogenic focus, polymorphic tachycardia, acute myocardial infarction, rupture of the atrium and/or coronary sinus, ventricular septal defect and sudden death. There is obviously much heat generated during extreme high voltage discharge.

Other methods that have been successfully used for ablation both in humans and animals, include the use of (a) comparatively low radio- frequency (500–700Khz) discharges via an endocardially positioned conductive electrode, (b) an intra-operative argon laser beam (c) cryoprobe to cool the tissue to sub-zero temperatures, (d) surgical dissection. Of these, radio-frequency discharge is now established as the method of choice for endocardial ablation of the A-V node and accessory pathways (q.v. Electrophysiology).

Further reading   Schechter DC, *Exploring the Origins of Electrical Cardiac Stimulation.* VII World Symp Cardiac Pacing, Vienna. Medtronic Inc., 1983.

ELECTROPHYSIOLOGICAL STUDIES

Study of the conductive disorders of the heart is usually performed in larger academic institutions where specialised equipment is available. Commonly known as *EPS, or EP studies*, the investigation requires conductive catheters to be introduced into the heart chamber(s) via a peripheral vein or artery. Once inserted:

(a) bipolar electrograms may be recorded from the distal electrodes at various sites where the electrodes are placed.

(b) they may also be used for stimulating or pacing of any site or chamber, or

(c) they may be required for sensing intrinsic or paced rhythms.

One of the most important recordable electrograms is that of the *HIS bundle (HBE)*. This low amplitude (less than 1 mV), medium frequency signal is recorded after placement of the electrode catheter against the ventricular septum in the region of the His bundle. Introduction may be via the antecubital or femoral vein, or less frequently, via the arterial system with the electrode catheter positioned in the non-coronary cusp of the aortic valve. Electrode catheters are also introduced into the high right atrium (HRA), low right atrium (HRA) and right ventricle (RV) respectively to record the high frequency components of the activity of each chamber. From these simultaneous recordings the physician is able to determine A-H (atrial to His) and H-V (His to ventricle) intervals. These timing periods are usually measured from recordings at paper speeds of 100 or 150 mm/sec. Together with scalar ECG leads they give much information of impulse formation and conduction anomalies .

FIGURE 99

A recording taken during an electrophysiological study showing the His bundle electrogram (arrowed) taken simultaneously with the atrial (A) and ventricular (V) electrograms. The upper two recordings are ECG limb leads.

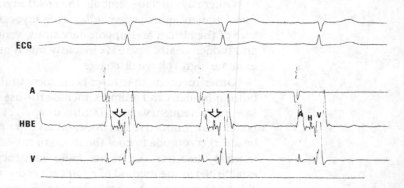

THE ELECTRODES

Unlike the pacing electrodes that are used for temporary pacing of the heart, EP electrodes are usually multi-polar, have good transference properties, distinct tip shapes that make them easier to position, and afford stability once they are introduced. Like the temporary pacing electrode they are radio opaque, made of a Dacron weave with a gum elastic cover that has an anti-thrombogenic coating.

The tip configuration is all-important for stable siting and like all other catheters used in cardiology, most are known either by brand names or after the name of the physicians who designed them (Zucker, Josephson, Myler, Damato, Cournand etc.). All have 2.5 mm male proximal connectors that may be inserted into a female extension box and /or amplifier. Description of the electrode catheter is sometimes described in the order of:

1. Name of the designer or the brand name,

2. Number of poles or electrodes at its distal tip,

3. Intended use,

4. French size and length in centimetres.

As an example:

1	2	3	4
Josephson	Quadpolar	Mapping electrode	6F × 110 cm

Let us now simply consider some of the ways that this technique can help the physician to diagnose conduction disturbances:

❑ From the scalar ECG P wave we are able to measure P-A interval corresponding to the intra atrial conduction time. It is measured from the onset of the P wave to the first part of the rapid high frequency component of the right atrial electrogram as shown on the HBE tracing. The normal range is 27 ± 18 ms.

❑ By recording electrograms from two sites of the right atrium i.e high (HRA) and low (LRA), antegrade or retrograde conduction may be determined. During antegrade conduction the HRA tracing would precede the LRA. The reverse would apply should retrograde conduction be present.

❑ The A-H interval gives a good indication of the conduction time through the AV node. It is measured from the first high frequency component of the LRA electrogram, which is physically close to the AV node, to the onset of the HBE. The normal range is 92 ± 38 ms. It is important that during the final positioning of the His electrode, the LRA-H duration be short. A lengthened LRA-H interval may indicate a poor position close to the right bundle.

❑ The H-V interval is the time taken for the impulse to reach the Purkinje network. It is measured from the onset of the His bundle deflection to the earliest deflection of the ventricular electrogram (V). The normal range is 43 ± 12 ms. A shortened H-V interval may also indicate a right bundle placement.

Imagine a tachyarrhythmia of unknown origin, one that may be either SVT or VT. By noting the timing of the His in relationship to the atrial and ventricular electrograms, it is possible to determine whether the impulse originates above, at, or below the His bundle. Other techniques include stimulation or pacing and/or sensing of either the atria or ventricles to determine the presence of abnormal pathways, such as those found in the Wolff-Parkinson-White syndrome. (Figure 100).

Summing up, the various standard procedures of an EP study will allow much information to be gained. These include:

❑ Retrograde conduction.

❑ The Sinus Node Recovery Time (SNRT). the time taken for the node to recover after prolonged rapid atrial overdrive pacing.

❑ The Sino-atrial Conduction Time (SACT).

FIGURE 100
X-ray taken during an EP study showing four catheter electrodes within the (i) high right atrium, (ii) right ventricle, (iii) coronary sinus and (iv) against the His bundle respectively. All were introduced via the right femoral vein.

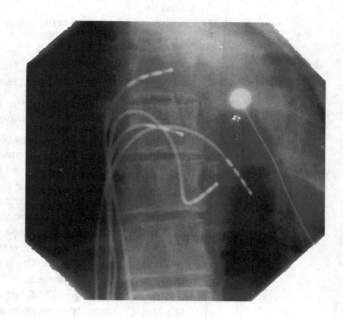

❑ Corrected Sinus Node Recovery Time (CSNRT) . The spontaneous sinus cycle length minus the SNRT. (less than 500 ms).

❑ AV Nodal conduction.

❑ His-Purkinje conduction.

❑ The determination and/or evaluation of the presence of accessory pathways, intra-atrial reentry, atrial flutter and fibrillation, AV nodal dysfunction, bradycardia, inducibility of ventricular tachyarrhythmias, the causes of syncope, etc.

The recording equipment In order to measure the His bundle electrogram and to compare its timing intervals to those of the right atrium and ventricle, it is necessary to use high gain amplifiers that will allow the internal electrograms to be more clearly defined. This is done by electronically filtering each signal within a specific bandwidth of 30–400 Hz.

Cardiac mapping Mapping is the technique of recording electrograms from the endocardial or epicardial surface of the heart in order to study cardiac activation potentials during arrhythmias. It is also used to locate arrhythmogenic foci with a view of ablation.

Endocardial mapping is performed in the catheterisation laboratory with the use of *catheter electrodes* that are inserted via the superficial veins. These electrodes are manually controlled in vitro by the operator in the same manner as cardiac catheters are manipulated.

Epicardial mapping is an intra-operative technique requiring open heart surgery. A multi-channel recorder is used with as many as over 100 sensors in contact with the heart, each connected to associated amplifiers. Without the aid of a computer, the technique of measurement analysis is time consuming.

It is of course, possible to map the heart with a single hand held probe which requires the time consuming task of the surgeon having to manually move the probe from one point of the heart to another, each time recording the electrogram underlying the probe. The flat distal end of the probe consists of three 0.5 mm dia. electrodes spaced at the corners of an equilateral triangle of 1mm sides. Another probe that is less frequently used is the finger probe. This type, shaped like a finger ring has a similar electrode pattern. It is worn around the middle finger and used for mapping inaccessible inferior areas of the heart surface.

Band electrodes are very useful for locating accessory pathways, as for example, in WPW syndrome. The placing of an elastic narrow cloth 'band', on which is mounted some 24 pairs of evenly spaced electrodes, around the AV groove and recording the electrograms from each of the areas where the electrodes are in contact with the heart, would, when measured against reference electrograms, give the location of the abnormal pathway.

FIGURE 101
The sock electrode
With kind permission of
Bard Electrophysiology

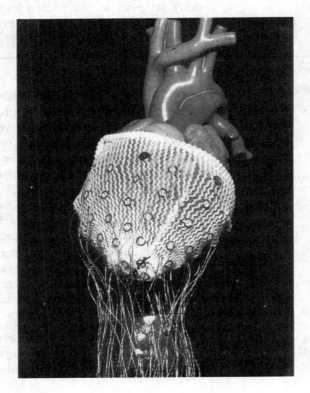

The *sock* electrode is a cloth mesh that is fitted over the lower portion of the heart. The ventricles are 'placed within it'. The interior surface of the sock consists of many evenly spaced button electrodes that are individually wired to amplifier channels of the physiological recorder. Analysis of the simultaneous recordings from all electrodes will reveal the origin or focus of a natural or provoked tachyarrhythmia.

Other electrodes used for mapping include patch types that may be placed upon specific areas of the myocardium and balloon electrodes that have multiple button electrodes situated on the exterior surface. The balloon is inserted and inflated within the ventricular chamber from where electrograms are recorded. Like the sock electrode, each button electrode is individually wired to amplifier channels.

Although the technique of cardiac mapping has virtually remained stagnant during the past twenty years, it has undergone many changes during the past few years. This can only be attributed to the advances of computer technology that have taken place. Not only is mapping time greatly reduced and therefore risks to the patient minimal, the computer is able to analyse intervals and allow the retrieved information to be quickly converted into an isochrone map. The patient's medical and personal data can be quickly reviewed and/or retrieved at any time, and storage of important data can be made on video tape.

RADIO-FREQUENCY (RF) ABLATION

The use of radio frequencies as a means of relieving muscular pain (shortwave diathermy) and for cutting and coagulation of tissue (cautery) has contributed, for many years, to the areas of physical medicine and surgery. During recent years its use has extended into the field of cardiology[62, 63] and is now a well established safe technique[64] for the ablation of conduction pathways within the heart, e.g. the atrioventricular node/His junction for the termination of AV nodal reentrant tachycardia (the most frequent type of paroxysmal supraventricular tachycardia) and the accessory pathways of Wolff-Parkinson-White syndrome.

Although direct current catheter ablation (DC shock), as described in the previous section, has been used with limitations over the past ten years, much concern had been shown regarding its safety and today few laboratories are using the technique.

Why radiofrequency? Radio-frequency ablation has many advantages when compared to DC ablation as shown in the following table, although one negative aspect of both methods is the occasional difficulty to visualise the

ECG immediately after (DC) or during (RF) the application of ablation current. DC shock distributes a large electrical field that causes the ECG to drift whilst radio-frequency will often be superimposed upon the ECG, each preventing immediate interrogation of the ECG signal. High frequency electrical filtration will often diminish the baseline artefact that RF produces. A pulse monitor used in conjunction with the electrocardiogram may therefore be advised.

Perhaps the only disadvantage of RF ablation is the comparatively small lesion it produces. This necessitates precise catheter placement and a stable electrode contact with the tissue.[65]

	DC shock	RF
1. Voltage	Large (500–3500)	small (40–60)
2. Frequency	1Hz (capacitive discharge)	500–750 kHz
3. Power (watts)	very large (± 60 000)	small (± 30)
4. Lesion size	large	small
5. Thoracic excitation	pronounced	none
6. General anaesthesia	yes	no
7. Barotrauma	yes	no
8. Patient risk	moderate/severe	minimal

What are radiofrequencies? Radiofrequencies are electromagnetic waves that cover the range of 10 kHz to over 10^6 MHz. i.e. 10 000 to 1 000 000 000 000 Hz and are used extensively for local and global communication. They may be transmitted through the ether or, if within the low range of the spectrum, via conductive cables. Very high frequencies, in the MHz band, are difficult to confine when conducted through electric cables, due to their reactive components that are generated. These reactive phenomena present capacitive and inductive interferences that may easily induce dangerous electric currents into nearby conductive cable or equipment. Low frequencies, i.e. below 100 kHz, on the other hand, cause stimulation of nerves and muscles.

For electrosurgical use, and that includes ablation techniques, mid-range frequencies of 500–750 kHz are used.

It must be remembered that radiofrequencies, when conveyed through a cable, will generate a radiating electromagnetic field that may readily be induced into other electrical circuits that are in close proximity. Cables carrying RF currents should therefore not be positioned parallel to other electrical cables, irrespective of the insulation qualities of either cable. It is well known that radiofrequencies whether transmitted through space or cable may be affected by external influences and the behaviour pattern of their distribution is sometimes confusing and bizarre.

The source The alternating current frequency used for RF ablation is obtained from a standard commercially available ablator that will allow the operator to control both temperature rise at the ablation site and the impedance generated between the electrodes. A standard *electrosurgical unit (ESU)* may also be used that will produce a frequency that is low in the RF spectrum.

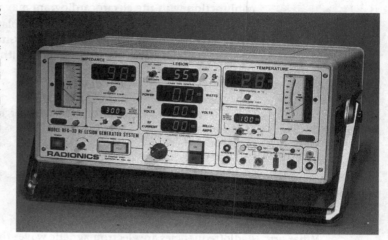

FIGURE 10.2
A commercial radio-frequency generator suitable for ablation of accessory pathways and abnormal ectopic foci allowing operator control of impedance and temperature during the procedure. With kind permission of Radionics, Burlington, USA.

When such frequencies are passed through tissue, resistive heat is generated. The amount of heat being dependent upon (*a*) the delivered energy, (*b*) size of the electrodes and (*c*) the electrode contact. When used for the relief of muscular pain, (shortwave or medical diathermy) frequencies within the 26 MHz band are used that operate at around 200 W of power. The heat generated is capacitive or inductive in nature. Large electrodes are usually used which dissipate the energy (and therefore heat) between the area contained within two large electrodes located on the body. Because the current density of the electrodes is low, heating of the tissue is never sufficient to cause necrosis. This type of radio-frequency generator cannot be used for electrosurgical or ablation use.

However, during electrosurgery, or surgical diathermy as it is sometimes known, a generator that produces a much lower frequency range is used (500–750 kHz) at a power of 60–200 W. A large indifferent electrode is positioned at some suitable site (buttocks, rear upper leg, etc.) and a small handheld probe used as an active electrode. The radio-frequency energy passes from the small active probe, where there is a very high intensity of power, to the indifferent electrode, so producing high resistive heat intensity at the site of the probe. Where the energy is dissipated over the large surface area of the indifferent electrode very little or no heat is produced. One can generally conclude that temperature is (*a*) inversely related to the size of the active probe, and (*b*) directly related to the power and the duration of discharge.

Electrosurgical Units operate in a mono or bipolar configuration and have three distinct power outputs:

1. *Cut* which is an abbreviation for cutting, will produce a continuous sinusoidal waveform that provides electric sparking producing smooth cutting. In practice, the tissue is not cut but heated so rapidly (desiccation) that the cells explode into steam that dissipates the heat produced.
2. *Coag*, an abbreviation for coagulation, produces an interrupted sinusoidal waveform that provides fulguration with minimum cutting. The effect is to reduce the tissue to carbon.
3. *Blend or mix* provides various degrees of cutting with haemostasis.

For ablation techniques the cutting output is more generally used providing a continuous sinusoidal waveform. Because the probe is blunt, unlike an electrosurgical blade, it desiccates the tissue. The control of the heat rise is considered a very important factor during ablation techniques. Figure 103 shows *Cutting* — the electrode is separated from the tissue, creating sparks that boil the tissue. *Fulguration* — causes long sparks that coagulate and necrose. *Desiccation* — the electrode remains in contact with the tissue causng deep coagulation. The effect of the discharge current depends upon (*a*) the power output, (*b*) the type of output i.e. bi or uni-polar (*c*) the ratio of the peak voltage to the RMS voltage , commonly known as the crest factor and (*d*) the waveform of the frequency component (damped, unmodulated or sinisoidal).

FIGURE 103
The three operative modes of the electrosurgical unit (ESU)

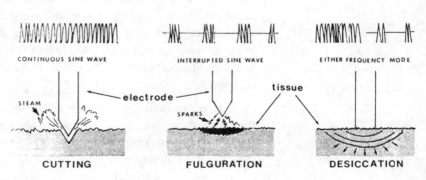

CONTINUOUS SINE WAVE   INTERRUPTED SINE WAVE   EITHER FREQUENCY MODE

tissue

STEAM — electrode — SPARKS

CUTTING   FULGURATION   DESICCATION

Method After the patient has been informed of the procedure, monitoring electrodes placed and an indifferent electrosurgical electrode positioned (left scapula, buttocks), a suitable transvenous steerable electrode (Mansfield/Webster, Medtronic) is introduced with its tip located at the necessary site for ablation. Once positioned, connection is made, usually via a switch box, to the Ablator or ESU output.

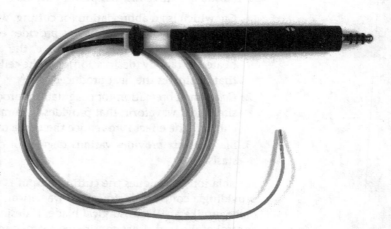

It is important that the operator be familiar with the instruction manual provided with the Unit and be aware of all suggested safety precautions. Detailed positioning of the catheter, the recommended output of the electrosurgical unit and the length of time of ablation have been well described.[66, 67, 68]

Lesion size is not solely related to power output or time duration but is also influenced by the electrode size, i.e. area of the distal tip. This electrode/tissue interface area may enhance the efficacy of radio-frequency ablation of the atrioventricular junction.[69] The larger the electrode area, the larger the lesion and the less likely that temperature rises will occur. Also given the same power, the less likely of ablation. As with most scientific applications there is much compromise.

It is unfortunate that any rise of temperature above 100° C at the electrode tip will cause a pronounced impedance rise between the active (catheter) and the indifferent electrodes. This rise of temperature is influenced by:

(*a*) The output, which if too high will cause the collection of coagulum (a sticky partially coagulated substance) and/or

(*b*) The interface contact, which will allow carbon to be deposited on the electrode tip caused by fulguration.

Both result in failure.

7 *Ultrasound Imaging*

This resumé is intended to cover some of the fundamental technical aspects of echocardiography and the student is well advised to consult some of the many excellent publications[70, 71, 72] regarding the medical applications of this exciting and involved diagnostic technique.

WHAT IS ULTRASOUND?

Ultrasound is sound waves above the audible range of frequency i.e. greater than 20 000 Hz, and similar to audible sound it propagates in a *longitudinal* manner i.e. it dissipates energy in the same direction as the motion of the molecules or particles. (*transverse* waves e.g. those that operate within the radio frequency band and travel at the speed of light, dissipate their energy at right angles to the motion of the particles).

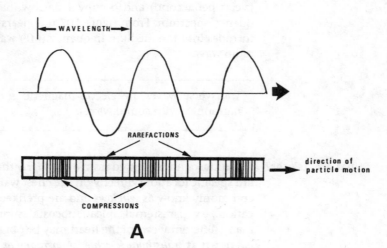

Figure 105A illustrates how the ultrasound energy particles become *compressed* (maximising pressure) and *rarefied* (minimising pressure) as the peaks and troughs of the frequency wave change.

Such sound waves are capable of penetrating tissue and behaving in a similar manner to light waves in that they may be transmitted, absorbed, reflected and refracted.

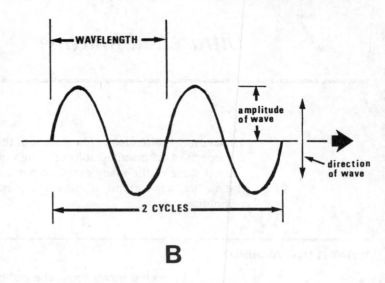

FIGURE 105B
The transverse propogation of particles that move at right angles to the direction of energy dissipation.

B

It is this ability of the ultrasound wave to be reflected from the various structures of the heart that allows the construction of a moving image to be displayed on a TV monitor. From this image diagnostic information is obtained. Although there is no defined upper limit, the frequencies used for the medical diagnostic application of ultrasound range between 2 and 10 MHz (2–10 million cycles per second) and occupy a narrow 'bandwidth' in the frequency spectrum. From figure 107 it appears that this bandwidth intrudes into the medium frequency (MF) waveband of transverse radio waves..

> Transverse waves are electro-magnetic and therefore cannot harmonise with sound waves.

What are its uses? The ultrasound is emitted from a *transducer* that is applied at standard specific locations directly on the chest wall. These locations are commonly know as *windows* and are prefixed by the site of application., e.g. parasternal, apical, subcostal, suprasternal, etc., so that many different views of the heart may be obtained. This technique is known as *transthoracic echo-cardiography or TTE*. The transducer may also be incorporated within a fibre optic gastroscope that is introduced into the oesophagus, so providing a high quality additional view, or window, of the heart This technique is known as *transoesophageal echocardiography* or *TEE*.

In addition to imaging, ultrasound is also used to measure the velocity of moving red blood cells within the circulation according to Doppler principles, and in this way the measurement of blood flow and pressure may be made (see later).

To better understand the behaviour of sound waves we must discuss the relationship between velocity, frequency and wavelength.

$$\text{Wavelength} = \frac{\text{Velocity}}{\text{Frequency}}$$

where:

❑ *Wavelength* is the longitudinal distance expressed in metres from one compression wave cycle to the next corresponding wave. The longer the wavelength the lower the frequency.

❑ The *velocity* of sound waves measured in metres/second is related to the molecular density, or compressibility of the medium through which it passes and also the temperature of the medium. Substances with high densities will transmit sound at higher velocities and lesser compressions.

For example, sound travels three times faster though lead than it does through copper. It travels through water at 1480 m/s and through air at 330 m/s.

However, the velocity that sound waves propagate through the soft tissues of the body is approximately 1 540 m/s and through bone considerably higher at 2600–4000 m/s.

❑ *Frequency* refers to the number of cyclic compressions that occur within a specific time period. The unit in which it is measured is the Hertz (Hz) and is equal to one cycle/second.

From the formula above the wavelength of the ultrasound wave that would be generated by a 2.5 MHz source may be determined.

$$\frac{\text{Velocity}}{\text{Frequency}} = \frac{1\ 540}{2\ 500\ 000} = 0.000616 \text{ metre or } 0.6 \text{ mm}$$

whereas that of a 5.00 MHz, 7.5 MHz and 10.0 MHz source would be 0.30 mm, 0.20 mm and 0.15 mm respectively. It is this inverse relationship between frequency and wavelength that determines the resolution, or the definition of the final echo.

Unlike radio waves that penetrate further into the atmosphere as the frequency is increased, ultrasound waves of higher frequencies (short wavelengths) do not penetrate well within the soft tissues of the body.

Frequencies ten times or more than those accepted for medical application would give very good resolution but would not penetrate body tissue. Generally, the shorter the wavelength (higher

FIGURE 106
The reflection and refraction as sound waves encounter an interface and are refracted as they pass through a second medium

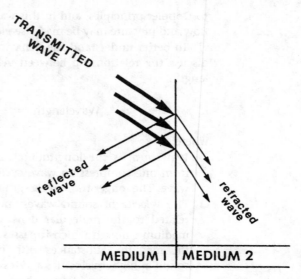

FIGURE 107
The frequency/wavelength spectrum of sound and electro-magnetic waves. The range indicated within the horizontal arrows are in the radio bandwidth.

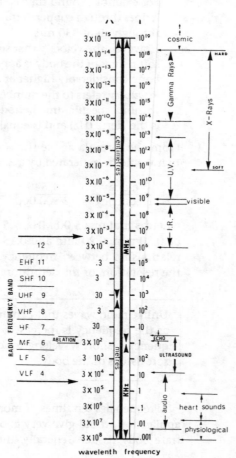

frequency), the better the resolution, although at higher frequencies absorption is increased causing less penetration. Transducers that operate at the higher range of 5.0–7.5 MHz are therefore more effectively used in small children who have thin chest walls. Transducers that operate at the lower frequencies of 2.00–3.5 MHz (longer wavelength), offer greater penetration at the expense of poor resolution. They are most commonly used for adults and especially for those patients who are obese or have barrel-chests.

Resolution is measured in millimetres and is the ability to identify two objects that are in close proximity to each other. If the two objects are 1mm apart then the system is said to have a resolution of 1mm. If they need to be 3 mm apart before being identified then the resolution is 3 mm.

HOW ARE ULTRASOUND WAVES GENERATED?

The unique properties of certain asymmetrical organic substances such as quartz, Rochelle salt (sodium potassium tartrate), tourmaline, barium titanate, lead zirconate when cut to specific shapes, are an essential part of the ultrasound system. These substances are known as Piezo-electric crystals and will expand in one direction and compress in the opposite direction when subjected to an alternating electric field. Conversely, when they are mechanically bombarded and compressed they will generate a charge on its surface as an electric voltage. Each piezo-electric crystal has its own resonant frequency and when an oscillating electric current is applied to it, it will mechanically distort and vibrate at the exact applied frequency. By sandwiching the crystal between two electrodes and applying an alternating sinusoidal current to the electrodes within the range desired, the crystal will emit ultrasonic waves. When these sound waves are *echoed or reflected* back to the crystal they cause the crystal to vibrate and produce minute electrical voltages that are within the range of *radio frequencies (RF)*, These voltages are then amplified and transformed into an image onto an oscilloscope or video display. It is these properties that are used to create the frequency *emitted* by the crystal and to analyse the reflected waves it *receives*.

Why do we use such high frequency ultrasound? It must be remembered that sound waves generated from any source will disperse in a radial fashion and become weaker in intensity to the square of the distance from the source. The returning echo to the transducer will also be considerably dispersed.

Ideally it would be of great advantage if the sound waves emitted from a transducer could be focussed and directed straight to the area that is under investigation, thus concentrating the energy to one specific point. This would create a comparatively larger echo from the heart with lessened dispersion. The important criterion is of course, the wavelength. It would be of no use generating an ultrasound signal having a wavelength that is longer than the distance from the transducer to the object being imaged.

Let us consider the following extreme example to elucidate this point:

Imagine a transducer that has a frequency of 25 000 Hz, just beyond audible sound. When applied to body soft tissue, the wavelength would be 1540 divided by 25 000, approximately 60 mm, far beyond the distance to the heart structure (1540 m/s being the propagation velocity through soft tissue). In order to allow time for the ultrasound wave to be discharged from the source and to be reflected back to the transducer, the wavelength must be very short compared to the distance it has to travel. This requires the use of a high frequency.

Other factors that are inter-related to the chosen frequencies include focussing, absorption, scatter and resolution.

The frequency at which the transducer operates will also affect its *near field* or fresnel zone, which is the distance that the emitted ultrasound beam will remain parallel before diverging to the *far field* or Fraunhofer zone. This distance is a function of (*a*) the radius of the transducer and the wavelength at which it operates. The shorter the wavelength and the larger the transducer, the longer the near field .

FIGURE 108
The effect of transducer radius to near and far field lengths

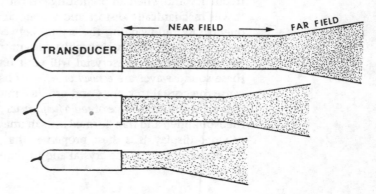

The divergent far field may also be minimised by the use of a transducer with a concave face or an acoustic lens which will narrow the ultrasonic beam and therefore increase its intensity at the focal zone.

Another method in which the ultrasound beam may be focussed is to use a transducer with multiple elements instead of a single one. Each of these elements may then be excited electroni-

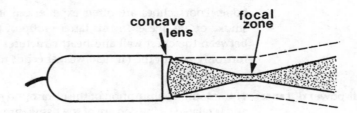

FIGURE 109
The increase of intensity and lessening of the far field divergence by use of a concave lens

concave lens

focal zone

cally in a timed sequential fashion. Depending upon the number of elements and the method of excitation it is possible to vary the focal zone and create a dynamically focussed ultrasonic beam.

Pulsed emission If the transducer were to continually emit ultrasound, one can imagine the jumble of artefact that would return to the transducer. Some reflected waves returning from anterior interface surfaces would arrive in a shorter time than those from middle and far distance surfaces. In order to overcome this, the ultrasound waves are emitted as a series of pulses. For a very short time the crystal, or *transducer* as it is commonly known, is excited by an oscillating current (usually between 500 and 2500 Hz/sec.) known as the *pulse repetition frequency* (PRF), causing it to emit pulsed ultrasound.

When the transducer is applied to the body it will deliver pulsed sound waves at the same frequency as the applied current that excited it. In between these very short bursts, part of the discharged energy in the form of a *reflected* wave returning from a *tissue interface* will cause the crystal to generate an electric current (a tissue interface is a boundary level at which point there is a change of acoustic density). The time required to travel the round-trip distance from the discharge of the sound wave to its returning echo should control the timing of the series of pulses emitted by the transducer so avoiding artefacts produced by a non-pulsed beam.

Unfortunately, this time, known as the *propagation velocity* is not constant throughout the trip as the interfaces have varying levels of *acoustic impedance,* some absorbing more of the sound than others. In fact no matter what kind of material the echo rebounding surface is composed of, some of the sound energy will be absorbed in the same way as audible sound is absorbed by an acoustic tile, rug or a curtain, as a result of the spongelike characteristics of the material. When sound waves enter they bounce around until they have lost much of their energy which, during the process, is transformed into heat.

Ultrasound actually reflects poorly from most tissue, as seen by the ratio of energy transmitted and received by the transducer, proving that much of the energy is absorbed e.g. it will not be reflected from air within lung or bowel, NOR will it easily penetrate bone. Poor echoes are often experienced in those patients who smoke or are obese. In this latter group of patients the distances between the chest wall and heart structures are greater and therefore only permit the far field weaker echos to be reflected.

Half-power distance

The amount of absorption of the ultrasound wave is extremely high and is related to the density of the tissue through which it traverses.

In ultrasound technology the term half power distance is sometimes used. This is the distance that half the original energy or intensity of the ultrasound beam is absorbed in its attempt to pass through a medium.

The table below shows the great variation of half power distances encountered within body tissue which accounts for much of the poor resolution experienced when recording from some patients. Note how well water allows ultrasound to pass compared to air. It is fortunate that within the soft tissues of the body the velocity of sound remains relatively constant, which allows accurate timing and depth to be measured

Half power distances measured in centimeters, and substances important in echocardiography. (Feigenbaum H. *Echocardiography*. Lea & Febiger, 3rd Edition. 1981.)

Water	380
Blood	15
Soft tissue	5 to 1
Muscle	1–0.6
Bone	0.7–0.2
Air	0.08
Lung	0.05

Remember — when recording the echocardiogram:

❏ Because air, or any gaseous medium, does not allow ultrasound to pass, there should be a positive contact between the transducer and the body surface by means of an ultrasound gel (not-KY jelly, ECG cream, Vaseline or defib paste).

❏ As previously mentioned, sound waves obey the laws of reflection and refraction and can be directed as a beam. This means that at right angles to the object being imaged the strongest echos will be received i.e. at a zero degree angle. Oblique signals will ᵇₑ reflected obliquely and returned at a much diminished strength.

❏ Near field echos that are returned from the anterior surface of the heart will produce much larger signals than those far field reflected from posterior and distant surfaces. The operator is able to equalise this inconsistency by a technique known as *time gain compensation(TGC)* that will allow the far field echos to be greater amplified than those reflected closer to the transducer. *depth compensation* controls will also allow the operator to vary the gain at any point of the recording.

FIGURE 110
The simplified circuit of the echocardiograph machine

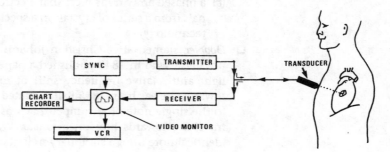

In figure 110 the *transmitter* is the unit that delivers pulsed signals to the crystal of the transducer causing it to discharge ultrasound. The *receiver* amplifies the weak ultrasound signals it receives from the transducer and relays these signals to the video monitor. Permanent recordings may be stored onto a video cassette recorder (VCR) or to a chart recorder. The *synchroniser (SYNC)* controls the operation of the transmitter and co-ordinates the timing frequencies of the video monitor.

THE EXAMINATION

There are several modalities that are used when imaging the heart. Each serves a different purpose but they are often all utilised in coming to a final diagnosis of the condition of the patient.

❑ *M-mode* (motion mode) echo is a single dimension vertical movement of echo waves along a single sound beam that are related to time.

❑ *Two-dimensional or 2D* imaging allows the heart to be viewed in real time in two dimensions using multiple echo beams that are displayed within an arc or sector. This may be more clearly understood if one were to imagine a single beam transducer that is held at right angles to the chest wall. By oscillating the transducer forwards and backwards within an arc, a two dimensional image (actually consisting of a series of one dimensional images) would be obtained.

Such a sector of ultrasound can be achieved using:

(a) a transducer that consists of multiple crystals arranged in a linear fashion. This type of transducer is not commonly used

(b) a mechanically operated oscillating transducer that utilises an electric motor to oscillate the transmitting crystal, or

(c) a phased array transducer that electronically discharges signals from a series of crystals in a specific order (phased array technology).

❑ *Doppler*, named after Christian Johann Doppler, an Austrian physicist, who in 1843 published a paper on the behaviour of light and relative frequency shift of moving stars travelling towards the earth. In 1845 Ballot related the Doppler principle to the single note of a trumpet that was played by a musician travelling towards him on a railcar. When compared to the identical note from a stationary musician he noticed a distinct difference in frequency, commonly known today as a *frequency shift*. This same principle is used to measure the velocity of blood as it flows through a vessel or orifice.

❑ *Contrast echocardiography.* By injecting a fluid such as saline, indocyanine green or blood into a peripheral vein, very small microbubbles can be seen on the echo screen traversing the right heart chambers and then absorbed within the lung. Although not strictly a routine part of the examination, combined with 2D imaging, is used to identify right to left intracardiac shunts, by the appearance of bubbles within the chambers of the left heart.

❑ *Colour flow imaging* is really a method of displaying Doppler ultrasound in a two dimensional format by superimposition on a 2D image. Combined with 2D imaging, Fourier filter transformation and the use of a sensitive colour processor the direction of forward and reverse blood flows can be shown in colour.

For timing purposes the ECG is simultaneously recorded during these ultrasound procedures and additional channels are often available for the recording of the phonocardiogram.

THE M MODE

The first echocardiograph machines were able to produce only one dimensional recordings of distance from the transducer to the structure of the heart being measured. They were amplitude measurements known as *A mode* recordings, that were later presented as *B mode*, or 'brightness mode' recordings in which the spot on a cathode ray tube increased its brightness proportionally to the amplitude of the receiving echo. By adding time as an additional dimension, these recordings became known as *M mode* or 'motion mode' and gave valuable information of movement of the various heart structures. The advanced machines of today use a cursor to automatically derive the M-mode echo from the two dimensional image.

FIGURE 111
The three common transducer angulations of M Mode recording

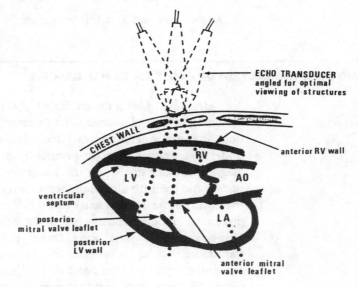

FIGURE 112
The M-mode echocardiograph showing movement of the anterior and posterior leaflets of the mitral valve (MVL). During systole both leaflets come tgether. CW — chest wall; RV — right ventricle; IVS — interventricular septum; ECG — electrocardiogram.

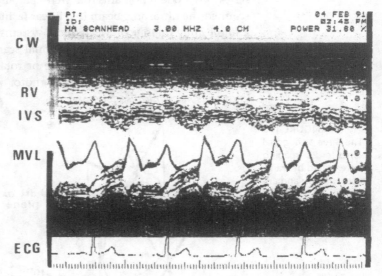

The three commonly used transducer positions as shown in figure 111 will measure the dimensions of the:

1. Right ventricular free wall, RV chamber (a guide to volume), motion and thickness of the ventricular septum (hypertrophy,

volume overload), LV chamber (volume), pericardial cavity (effusion) and fractional shortening (an index of function).

2. Mitral valve (mobility of the leaflets, mitral stenosis, non-compliant left ventricle).

3. Aortic valve and root and left atrium.

TWO DIMENSIONAL (2D) OR CROSS SECTIONAL IMAGING

A disadvantage of M mode recording is that it provides only a single dimensional view of the heart and therefore gives limited information of spatial orientation or lateral dimension of the structure under investigation. A major advance in the use of ultrasound as a diagnostic tool came when the transducer was able to scan the surface and transmit ultrasound waves through anatomic 'slices' of the organ, either in a *long axis* or *short axis* views, depending on the placement and directional rotation of the transducer on the chest. This was done in several ways. One of the early methods used a transducer that had a series of in-line multi-elements that were sequentially excited from one side to the other. It was in effect a series of B mode echograms that were spatially tracked. It moved or scanned the ultrasonic beam in a linear fashion and was known as a *linear array transducer.* Mechanical systems were also developed that allowed real time two dimensional scanning by causing the transducer beam to rapidly oscillate or rotate through an arc or sector by means of a small electric motor within it. These were known as *mechanical sector scanners.*

FIGURE 113
The three orthogonal planes for 2D imaging determined by transducer rotation and angulation

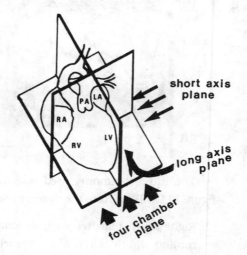

FIGURE 114
Typical orientations of the transducer that will obtain the three orthogonal planes (A) long, (B) short and (C) four chamber. (From Henry W et al. Circulation 62: #2 1980)

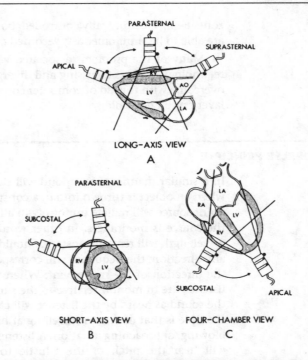

FIGURE 115

The apical long axis view of the four chambers of the heart. The point of the arc represents the transducer position on the chest wall. The two upper chambers are the ventricles and the two lower the atria.

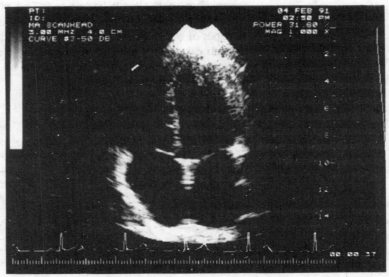

The most popular transducers are multi-element, electronically controlled, and able to scan at high speed a sector of some 80–90 °. These *phased array* or *real time sector scanners* have either a fixed focussed beam or dynamic focussing that provides a long focal zone. Being electronically controlled, both M mode and 2D images are able to be simultaneously recorded on the same monitor.

Many of the problems associated with ultrasound transducer technology, such as focussing and divergence or scatter have been overcome with the aid of computer controlled circuitry and multi-layer crystal technology.

THE DOPPLER PRINCIPLE

In a similar manner that a pond will ripple in a radiated fashion when an object is thrown into it, a constant sound emitted from a point source will radiate uniformly in all directions, assuming that the source is motionless. In other words, the frequency and the wavelength will remain constant. Should the point source move in any direction, the frequency will correspondingly increase towards the direction of the movement. When the source of sound, or a listener, are in motion relative to the surrounding air, the pitch of the sound as heard by the listener will change. The most common example is that of a train travelling at high speed with its whistle blowing, approaching a station. A listener standing on the station, will hear the pitch of the whistle to be higher as the train approaches than after it has passed. This change in frequency is commonly known as *Doppler shift* or Doppler effect and is seen in all types of waves when the source and listener are moving relative to each other. This change of frequency is directly related to the velocity of the mass and also the angle to which the listener is directed towards the source.

FIGURE 116

(A) The constant frequency and wavelength of a stationary sound source, illustrating how the sound radiates in all directions. (B) The increased lateral frequency and decreased wavelength at the front of a moving source travelling towards the listener.

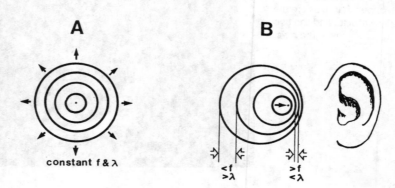

The Doppler effect is not confined to sound. Doppler originally described how the colour of a star was influenced by its movement away or towards the viewer. The wavelength difference caused the change in colour. A similar phenomenon occurs when underwater sound waves are reflected by a moving submarine (Sonar). During World War 2 Doppler technology was effectively used as long ago as 1941 as a means of detecting the presence of enemy aircraft (Radar).

The shift of frequency (and wavelength) is equated by the following formula:

$$\text{Doppler shift} = \frac{2FV.\cos @}{P}$$

where:

❑ F is the frequency emitted from the transducer.

❑ V is the velocity of the mass that is moving away from or towards the ultrasonic beam (blood).

❑ @ is the angle of incidence between the beam and the moving mass

❑ P is the propagation velocity of sound through biological tissue (1560 m/s).

The principle of Doppler as used in echocardiography for the measurement of blood flow and velocity has created a new dimension in the diagnostic capabilities of this technique. Combined with 2D imaging it allows the quantitation and detection of a host of cardiac anomalies that were originally confined to the invasive procedures of the catheterisation laboratory. Most shunt situations are detectable; valve areas are able to be measured; cardiac output may be indirectly quantitated by measurements of flow through the aortic valve and of the root of the aorta; the analysis of tricuspid regurgitation allows the estimation of right ventricular pressure to be made; pressure gradients across the aortic valve may be assessed, and a host of structural defects can also be determined.

FIGURE 117
The angle of incidence of the ultrasonic beam. See text.

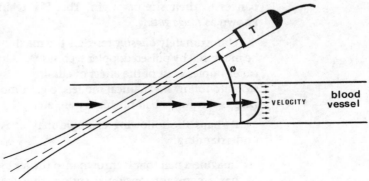

One major difference of technique between 2D imaging and Doppler is that in order to accurately measure the amount of Doppler shift and subsequent blood flow, the transducer beam must be parallel to the flow, whether it be antegrade or retrograde. This means the angle of incidence must be at 0 or 180 °. A transducer held at 90 ° to the flow would record no Doppler shift. Slight angulation of the transducer within the overall range of 30 °, i.e. 15 ° either side of the vessel, presents little error (less than 4 %) provided it remains within the limits of flow direction

Angulation over these limits entails much more elaborate mathematical quantitation as other considerations are introduced, for example; scatter, sensitivity and signal losses etc. It is often very difficult, and at times impossible, when imaging the heart to precisely angulate the transducer in the direction of blood flow. The Doppler shift is obtained from the direction of blood flow. From a midline on the oscilloscope an upward or *positive* direction usually indicates blood flow *towards* the transducer and a downward or *negative* indicates a flow *away* from the transducer. The velocity of blood flow being directly related to the doppler frequency shift.

Two distinct types of Doppler technology are used during cardiac imaging:

Pulsed wave doppler In pulsed wave doppler (PW) a single crystal transmits and receives the ultrasound signal. It is activated to produce a series of very short duration pulses at a selected frequency that are discharged in bursts from the transducer. Between these bursts no further signals are discharged until all returning echos are received and as ultrasound travels at 1560 m/s through body tissue, the time of its return can be accurately calculated as can the depth of its penetration. PW allows the velocity to be measured within a small range at a variable depth along the ultrasonic beam, and provides a high degree of *range resolution* that allows the operator to pinpoint flow disturbances to their site of origin. This PW technique is commonly known as *range gating*.

Unfortunately *aliasing* restricts the maximum velocity that can be measured by pulsed doppler techniques. Although many electrical examples exist of the effect of aliasing, it is more readily understood to follow mechanical models, e.g. in movie filming, carriage wheels turning, a ball hitting a wall, etc.

Perhaps the following example may assist the student in its understanding.

1. Imagine a ball that is thrown into the air by means of a bat that has a constant tensioned spring, that would deflect the ball vertically one metre each time the ball is returned to the bat.

The frequency that the ball is hit will depend upon the time it takes the ball to make the round trip from and to the bat.

2. Now let us replace the spring with a stronger one that has increased tension. This will allow the ball to be thrown higher in the air. It will also now take longer to return to the bat.

3. Therefore the frequency at which the ball is thrown by the spring would have to be decreased.

4. Should however, the throwing frequency of the spring remain the same, the ball would not be thrown as soon as it reached the spring, but would have to wait until the spring was ready for its next thrust.

It is this asynchronous relationship between the time travelled by the ball and its spring discharge frequency that limits the repetitive accuracy of the cyclic response.

In this simple analogy, imagine the ball to be the carrier of the *pulse*. The frequency at which the ball is thrown the *pulsed repetition frequency* (PRF), the height that the ball is thrown to be the *sample volume depth* and the returning ball to be the Doppler *shift*. Because the pulsed Doppler signal will not discharge until it has received the returning echoes from the previous pulse, it is unable to accurately measure high velocities as seen in some valvular stenotic lesions. In other words the maximum frequency shift is limited to one half of the Pulsed Repetition Frequency. It is this limitation known as the *Nyquist limit* that presents the returning echoes in a reverse direction whenever the blood flow velocity is greater than half the sampling rate. It is seen as 'wrapping around' itself and although the machine correctly determines the flow velocity it plots the flow on the wrong side of the zero line. Should the depth of the sample volume increase the PRF will decrease and a subsequent decrease in the maximum shift of frequency will occur.

FIGURE 118
The effect of aliasing (A) The unambiguous recording of continuous wave showing the corect maximum and minimum velocity. (B) The ambiguous recording of pulse wave. (C) The maximum and minimum doppler shift.[70]

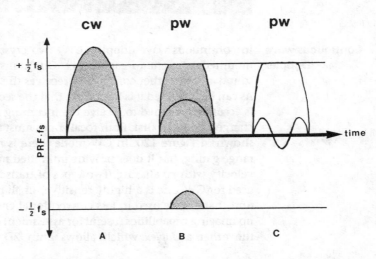

Figure 118 (B) illustrates the effect of frequency aliasing when using PW doppler, limiting the measurement of maximal velocity of blood flow (frequency shift). The peak of the frequency curve has been displaced to the negative portion of the graph. When moderate aliasing is seen, moving the baseline either up or down allows the operator to double the frequency display limits. This technique is known as *zero shifting* and eliminates the aliasing artefact. It does not, however, affect the limitations imposed by the Nyquist theory.

Figure 118 (C) shows the estimation of mean frequency, which is the average of both positive and negative parts of the spectrum for each instant of time. This estimation depends upon the spatial distribution of the intensity of the ultrasound beam and the velocity distribution of the source.

FIGURE 119
A CW Doppler recording of a regurgitant flow across the mitral valve

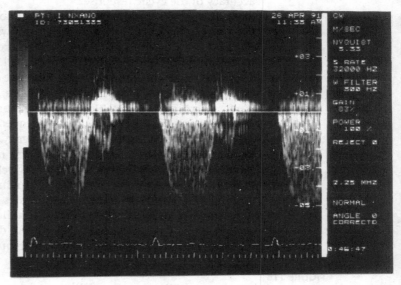

Continuous wave Doppler

In continuous wave doppler *(CW)* two crystals are used that are mounted adjacent to each other. One transmits bursts of ultrasound and the other continually receives the echoed information. As can be imagined it is important that the second receiving crystal is accurately aligned to receive the incoming signals that were discharged from the first. Both focal zones must therefore intercept as shown in Figure 120. In CW mode there is no *range resolution* or range gating, but it does provide unlimited measurable maximum velocity with *no* aliasing. Two types of transducers are commonly used for CW, one is a highly sensitive, small pencil type dedicated unit that can be used in less conventional chest windows and has no imaging capabilities (useful for assessment of valve lesions), and the other a *duplex* which allows both 2D and Doppler to be recorded. The advantage of range resolution (PW) and unlimited velocity measurements (CW) greatly enhance the usefulness of Doppler as a diagnostic tool.

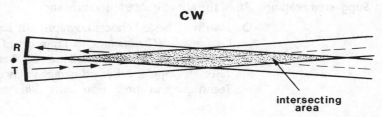

CW

R
•
T

intersecting area

FIGURE 120
The two crystals of the continuous wave transducer showing the intersecting area in which is contained the focal zone. R = Receiving T = Transmitting.

A further advancement in ultrasound technology is *real time 2D colour flow imaging (CFI)*. This spatial representation of blood flow allows colour to enhance the antegrade or retrograde blood flows and necessitates a powerful colour processor to carry out this function. The colours red and blue are used to display the mean direction and velocity. Usually, all shades of red indicates blood flow

Towards the transducer and all shades of blue away from the transducer. By introducing the colour green, variance of flow patterns whether laminar or turbulent, may be identified. The different colour densities or hues of red or blue represent the relative velocities (front cover showing moderate mitral regurgitation). It must be remembered that PW and CW Doppler displays and represents changes of velocity at the point of a single sampled volume (PW) or along a single scan (CW). Neither is able to display flow images nor to readily recognise turbulence unless there is spectral broadening. The method of determining the frequency changes i.e velocity, is known as Fourier Filter Transformation or FFT (q.v. Glossary).

The technique of colour flow does shorten the time of the echo examination and provides the operator with a colour picture or 'anatomical angiogram' of regurgitant valvular lesions, clearly showing on the 2D image the mean velocity and the direction of flow. This enables the operator to better angulate the transducer. Because the heart is a moving object, wall movements are often clearly displayed. (See example on cover jacket)

Stress echocardiography The American College of Cardiology has recommended (*Cardiology* April 1991) stress studies be undertaken in conjunction with echo analysis in those patients who:

- ❑ have a non-diagnostic treadmill stress ECG,
- ❑ have conduction abnormalities,
- ❑ are required to have any invasive intervention,
- ❑ are known to have high false-positive ECG changes or

❑ have undergone a myocardial infarction, and prognostic information is required

Suggested reading All of the above quoted literature and:

❑ Martin L, Basic Echocardiography. In Bronson L. *Textbook of Cardiovascular Technology* J.B. Lippincott Co., Phil. USA. 1987.

❑ Nishimura RA, Miller FA, Callahan MJ, Benassi RC, Seward JB & Tajik AJ. Doppler echocardiography: Theory, Instrumentation, Technique and application. *Mayo Clin Proc* 60: 321, 1985.

8 Electrical Safety

It is more than 35 years since the first reported incident of an electrocution occurred at the London Hospital of a patient undergoing surgery.[73] During the past two decades great advances have taken place in the design of medical equipment in order to reduce the risk of electrical shock to the patient. Most of these advances have today made it almost impossible for a patient to receive a lethal shock.

For example, the use of *optical isolators* has prevented a direct electrical communication between the monitoring apparatus and the patient - once a common cause of electric shock.

The use of radio-frequency *telemetry* to transmit physiological signals to the recording device obviates direct electrical connection to the patient.

Earth leakage detectors as wired in many home electrical supples disconnect currents above critical levels that may be conducted to ground via the patient.

Current limiting diodes disallow currents beyond their operating range to flow to the patient from monitoring devices.

The use of *isolated power supplies* using an isolation transformer prevents live currents flowing to ground via the patient.

By the use of an *isolated ground system* which separates the localised ground of the patient from the ground of the building (in a similar way that the isolation transformer separates two distinct circuits) prevents current flow through the patient.

Today many manufacturers are adopting *instrument isolation* as a means of shock protection, but to be effective all other equipment used within the area of the patient must also be isolated. Many diagnostic and therapeutic machines are *battery powered* which considerably reduce the risks.

Each of the methods is a compromise to ensure absolute safety and some have drawbacks when used in conjunction with other equipment. Some of the methods used to obtain electrical safety are expensive and often do not relate to the design of the specific piece of equipment, e.g. an isolated ground system should not interact with other services that may be grounded to water pipes and taps, gas lines and lighting conduits.

REMEMBER

Each individual piece may provide absolute protection. More than one may not. However, despite these technical advances and the better understanding of the risks of electric shock by most clinical personnel, circumstances do arise when the monitored patient is sufficiently compromised to the extent that his or her life may be in jeopardy. Many of these situations occur because the attending clinical personnel do not, or cannot, appreciate potentially harmful conditions or situations.

RISKS

Before detailing the conditions that place the patient at risk, it is important to realise that:-

❏ Man is very susceptible to electric shock,
❏ The opportunities of electric shock are greatly increased to the patient who is in contact with electrical instrumentation,
❏ The greater the number of electrical devices to which he or she is connected, the greater the risk.

Let us consider the patient who is admitted to a CCU having experienced an acute myocardial infarction. Such a shocked, exposed, perspiring patient could well be ECG monitored, have a temporary pacemaker electrode in situ, be intra-aortic balloon pumped, electronically ventilated with an attached humidifier and, have a flow-directed thermistor catheter inserted for the measurements of cardiac output.

Imagine also the patient who has returned to a post surgical ICU having undergone by-pass surgery who may have much of the above mentioned equipment attached plus suction drainage and perfused with the use of electronic controllers and pumps. Not only is there a risk of some of these devices allowing *leakage currents* to pass through the patients body but equally important is the risk of currents being *induced* from one electrical conductor to a sensor that is parallel and adjacent to the conductor. When two parallel electrical conductors are in close proximity, a capacitive coupling exists between them and a small quantity of electrical charge may be created through the insulation of one into the other.

CAUSE AND EFFECT

Death from electric shock is invariably due to cardiac arrest, whether it be standstill or ventricular fibrillation and is caused by any condition that will produce a *potential difference (p.d.)* between the heart and the source. The effect of the electric shock will depend on the *amount of current* that is allowed to flow and although this relationship has been well described many years ago by Dalziel[74,75,76], Burchell,[77] Starmer,[78] Whalen[79] and others, it is worthy of recollection.

As early as 1936 Ferris and co-workers carried out a comprehensive animal study at the Bell Telephone Laboratories at Columbia University, USA, to determine the currents required to produce ventricular fibrillation. Although these experiments were performed on dogs they did, when extrapolated, give indications to the effects on man.

The current densities and their effects listed below refer to voltages within the household power range (in the United States) and to shock delivered across the intact dermis.

- ❑ Threshold of perception: 0-10 milliamps
  This is the level of shock that is barely felt. i.e. when the hand is lightly moved against an electric conductor and a tingling sensation is felt.
- ❑ "Let-go" threshold: 10-16 milliamps.
  This is the point at which the subject is able to let go the conductor or appliance he is holding. Beyond that point he is unable to let go as the musculature of his hand vigorously contracts.
- ❑ Pain and fright: 16-20 milliamps
  Pain and fright are experienced beyond the let-go point.
- ❑ Sensation of heat, collapse, apnea: 20-50 milliamps
  either or all may occur.
- ❑ Possible ventricular fibrillation: 50-100 milliamps
- ❑ Ventricular fibrillation and death if untreated: over 100 milliamps.
- ❑ Burns: 2 amps and above
- ❑ Deep burns, body overheat: excessive high currents

The lower end of these ranges might well be accepted from power sources of higher voltages as used in Europe, South Africa, some South American countries and many other parts of the world.

FACTORS

How then, we may ask, is it possible for a potential difference (p.d.) to exist and what are the factors involved that cause electric shock to be harmful? They are four in number:-

1. *Electrical impedance.* Simply, this refers to the resistance to electrical current flow that the body imposes. Many years ago Freiberger[80] carried out tests on 2,600 corpses and 25 living volunteers to determine the electrical resistance of the body, i.e. hand to hand and hand to foot with intact dermis. He found,

as expected, that resistance to electrical flow varied with the applied voltage.

- At 30 volts the average resistance was found to be 10 000 ohms,
- At 100 volts it was 4 000 ohms,
- At 200 volts 2 000 ohms.

All these measurements were taken under normal dry skin conditions. At a potential of 250 volts the skin resistance would approximate 1800 Ohms and by Ohms law this would allow a current of 140 milliamperes to flow, enough to provoke ventricular fibrillation. With very dry skin the current flow might be reduced to much lower than 100 milliamperes. With a very moist skin the level could rise to 230 milliamperes.

2. *Electrical pathway* refers to the "entrance and exit" of the electrical source within the body. An important point to remember is that the chest is, at commercial frequencies i.e. 50 or 60 Hz, a volume conductor of electricity. This means that electrical current does not take a direct pathway through the upper portion of the chest should, for example a shock be received from hand to hand, but encompasses the whole chest, in which is contained the heart and lungs. Under these conditions it is not difficult to appreciate the risks of electric shock.

Let us consider another example. Should the fingers of one hand be connected to the live and neutral sockets of a power source and the subject be standing on an insulated floor, he would receive a painful non-lethal shock though the fingers that are in contact with the live and neutral sockets. However were he to place the finger of one hand into the live socket and a finger of the other hand into the neutral socket of the power source he would be at considerable risk, despite him standing on the insulated floor. In the first situation the pathway is between the fingers of one hand, and in the second situation from one hand to the other, crossing the chest.

Consider also the bird perched on a high tension power cable that is carrying some thousands of volts. It is quite safe as long as there is no pathway to ground or to any other conductor that will allow the current to pass through its body.

3. *Current density* or the amount of current flow per unit area, has a direct relationship to body impedance, and provided the voltage remains constant, is proportional to the risks. The higher the density the greater the risk of inducing ventricular fibrillation. Females usually have a lower skin resistance than males and caucasians a much lower resistance than negroids. The blonde light skinned female of the northern hemisphere would therefore be at a greater disadvantage to shock than her central African counterpart.

Body weight will also determine the effects of shock. The larger the body mass the greater the impedance to current flow and the moderately less likelihood of ventricular fibrillation.

4. *Shock duration* or the length of time an electric shock is administered has been shown to be related to the risks of ventricular fibrillation. Much of this work was carried out on dogs by Ferris, in 1936; Kiselev, in 1963; and Kouwenhoven, Johns Hopkins University, Baltimore in 1959 and later re-evaluated by Dalziel and Lee in 1968.[81]

The level of fibrillating current is inversely proportional to the square root of the duration of shock. This unusual relationship has been attributed to the complicated nature of ventricular fibrillation and might be related to multifocal origins of fibrillatory response.

Subdermal shock We have so far mentioned the effects of electric shock through the intact dermis where fibrillation is likely to be provoked by currents greater than 50 milliamperes. However a shock administered beneath the skin may be three times more lethal than one delivered through the skin.

Even more important:

A shock delivered directly to the heart is 5000 times more lethal. This means that an electrical current as low as 10-20 microamperes may provoke ventricular fibrillation should it be directed to the heart.

There are many instances when this can occur especially during cardiological diagnostic and therapeutic procedures that involve placing electrically conductive probes, catheters, needles, etc within the heart muscle or within one or more of the chambers. Most of these instances are usually associated to one of two causes:

Earth leakage

This term is used to describe the situation when an electrical device leaks current to ground. One may imagine using an electric iron, lightly touching the metal part and experiencing a tingling feeling. This feeling is due to a small amount of electric current from the "live" wire being dissipated to the chassis of the iron to the hand. Were the iron not grounded - and the live wire within the iron in contact with the chassis the shock might have been severe enough to create a density and pathway to cause fibrillation. In the clinical situation imagine a piece of ungrounded power-driven equipment to which is connected a conductive catheter positioned within the heart of the patient. This equipment might be an electrophysiological stimulator or pacemaker, or an ECG machine that is recording a pericardiocentesis or an intracardiac electrogram.

These situations become even more critical when current pathways are accidentally caused by medical staff.

Let us consider a few unusual but nevertheless, possible situations:

1. A patient is connected to an external pacemaker and monitored, lying on an *electrically operated motorised bed*. For some reason the frame of the metal bed is ungrounded, probably because the ground wire had become unattached within the power plug, or had broken within the cable after it had been run over many times by the bed wheels. During the life of the bed much dust would have congregated over the windings within the electric motor (a common occurrence of electric motors that generate static electricity when operating) allowing a small amount of current, that would normally have dissipated to ground via the intact ground cable, to leak to the metal frame of the bed.

   Now one of the clinical staff wishing to adjust the proximal portion of the electrodes of an external pacemaker, and who is sitting on the side of the bed, one hand touching the exposed proximal portion of the electrodes that are within the heart and the other hand touching the now "live" bed. The operator is not likely to feel any shock through his intact dermis (especially if the current is below perception levels) but he would act as a micro-current carrying conductor from the bed - through his body - to the pacemaker electrode - to the heart of the patient - and finally to ground via the ECG electrode located on the patients chest. Such a current may be enough to cause the patient to fibrillate.

2. *Pericardiocentesis* is the technique commonly used for the diagnosis of chronic and less commonly, acute pericardial effusion that is usually performed under x-ray guidance in a catheterisation laboratory or, under certain circumstances, echo guidance. A short bevel needle of 18g or larger is slowly introduced through the chest wall (sub-xiphoid or precordial) until its tip is made to contact the myocardium. Prior to introduction an exploring ECG electrode cable is connected to the hub of the needle by means of a sterile alligator clip cable. The ECG is monitored throughout. On contact of the tip of the needle with the heart, an injury pattern (S-T elevation) will immediately be seen on the recorded electrocardiogram (figure 121).

   Slow withdrawal of the needle will show the disappearance of the injury pattern signifying that the needle is within the pericardial cavity. Fluid is then aspirated into a syringe connected to the needle hub. The continuous handling of a metal conductor (needle) throughout this procedure may allow minute electric currents to flow directly to the heart from the operator OR leakage currents may flow from the ECG recording mechanism. Such currents may provoke arrhythmias. The alligator cable should always be connected to a Wilson ECG terminal or be isolated from an electrical source. .

NOTE

> Whenever conductive electrodes or needles that are within or in contact with the heart are manipulated, it is important that the operator wear rubber gloves

FIGURE 121
The electrocardiographic changes seen during entry and exit of the centesis needle.

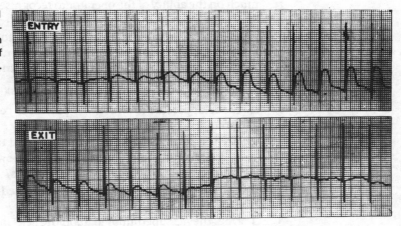

Two reliable methods exist that can prevent either of these hazardous situations:

❑ Isolation of the instrument chassis so that it is non-conductive or
❑ Ensure that the chassis is properly grounded. The former necessitates expensive constructional modifications involving the isolation of all components attached to the chassis, whilst the latter is a simple constructional design commonly used in combination with methods outlined.

Induction

When an electric current flows within a conductor an electromagnetic field is generated around the current carrying conductor. Should a second conductor be positioned in close proximity and parallel to the first and contained within its magnetic field, an electric current will be "induced" from the first into the second conductor and will flow within its circuit. This method of transference of electrical current should not be overlooked when many lines of cables are meant to run to equipment attached to the patient. The operator must be especially careful not to allow patient cables to be in close proximity to power cables or those carrying high frequency currents such as is used in electro-surgical equipment, i.e. cautery or diathermy.

REMEMBER

> Soft cable insulation does not prevent induction.

How can one be sure that the patient is well protected from the hazards of electric shock? The answer to such a question depends much on the ability of the operator to recognise causal situations.

Modern monitoring equipment as supplied by reputable manufacturing companies must by law comply to strict safety regulations and the circumstances whereby a patient receives an electric shock are usually due to lack of regular electrical maintenance.

The most important questions one should ask are:

❑ Is the apparatus to which the patient is connected isolated or grounded

❑ Are the power cable wires firmly attached to the plug?

❑ If grounded, is the ground pin of the power plug electrically connected to the chassis of the apparatus?

❑ Is there alternating current superimposed on the monitored ECG?

❑ Does the AC superimposed upon the ECG increase in amplitude whenever the patients skin is touched?

❑ When was the monitor last checked for leakage currents?

Alternating current interference may indicate that the patient is receiving an electric shock below the level of perception and should be investigated. Check that cables are not in close proximity to each other and that none are parallel or close to a power carrying conductor. Check the ECG electrodes, especially the ground connection. Are the electrodes dried out? These are a very important considerations, for without adequate grounding, it may be possible that leakage currents may easily flow through the patient. It is surprising that many hospitals, even large academic centres, do not carry out routine electrical checks of all electrically powered quipment that has connection to the patient.

A word about *static electricity* is appropriate at this point. This high voltage type of electric shock may be experienced by the hospital personnel or patient. It is a non-flow electrical charge that is caused to discharge to the patient and is best avoided by the control of humidity. Under normal circumstances it is felt when a metal conductor is touched and poses little hazard, but to the electrically susceptible patient who has, for example, an acute myocardial infarction, it is not only frightening, which may in itself precipitate a tachyarrhythmia, but may also interfere with other functional equipment to which the patient is attached. It is the kind of shock that is sometimes experienced when opening the metal handle of a car door.

Few other branches of hospital medicine rely so much on electronic instrumentation for diagnoses and treatment as cardiology and the technologist should always be aware of possible situations, sometimes disastrous, that can be caused when A.C. interference is seen to be superimposed on the monitored ECG. This is especially so when the electrocardiogram is used to control or trigger the operation of certain life support systems such as intra-aortic balloon pumps, pacemakers, cardiovertors or in specific instances during electrophysiological studies.

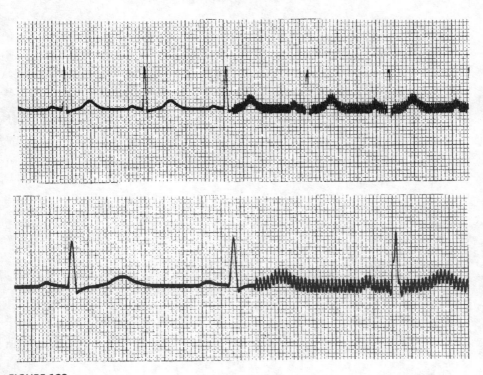

FIGURE 122

Alternating current power interference superimposed on the baseline of the electrocardiogram. The upper tracing is recorded at 25 mm/s and the lower at 50 mm/s. The interference oscillates at 50 Hz corresponding to the frequency of the alternating source. (In the United States, and certain other countries, the oscillations would be seen as 60 Hz)

Although the administration of an electric shock may not be physically felt the patient may be at a greater risk than believed, especially when there are many electrical devices connected and alternating current interference is present on the monitored electrocardiogram.

Suggested reading   Carr JJ & Brown JM. *Introduction to Biomedical Equipment Technology.* 2nd Ed. Prentice Hall. 1993.

Tables, Formulae, Calculations

Cardiovascular sizes of catheters and needles

French size	ID	OD	Needle gauge ID	Needle gauge OD
1.8F	0.28	0.61	20	23T
3F	0.36	1.00	20	23
4F	0.46	1.33	18	22
4FT	0.58	1.33	18	20T
5F	0.66	1.67	16	19
5FT	0.86	1.67	16	19T
6F	0.91	2.00	15	18
6FT	1.17	2.00	15	17T
7F	1.17	2.33	13	17
7FT	1.47	2.33	13	15T
8F	1.42	2.67	12	15
9F	1.63	3.00	—	14
9FT	1.98	3.00	—	13T

Cardiovascular sizes of catheters and needles are usually measured in French (size 1F = 0.33 mm), or needle gauge and are classified according to the outer diameter of the catheter or needle. The letter T indicates a thin-wall catheter or needle.

Arterial oxygen content of inspired gas at 1 and 2 atmospheres

	Air	O_2 1 Atmosphere	O_2 2 Atmospheres
Haemoglobin saturation %	97	100	100
Dissolved O_2 in plasma (ml/100 ml)	0.3	2.0	4.3
Total O_2 content (ml/100 ml)	0.85	21.0	23.3

Alveolar air partial pressures at 1 and 2 atmospheres

Alveolar pO2 mmHg	105	673	1433
Alveolar pCO2	40	40	40
Alveolar pN2	569	0	0
Alveolar pH	47	47	47

Normal partial pressures and pH of blood

	Arterial	Venous blood
pO2	90	40
pCO2	40	46
pH (plasma)	7.45	7.43
pH (corpuscles)	7.12	7.11

Abbreviations of some medical terms

Term	Latin	English
a.c.	ante cibum	before food
ad lib	ad libitum	to the desired amount
b.d or b.i.d.	bis in die	twice daily
o.m.	omni mane	each morning
o.n.	omni nochte	each night
p.c.	post cibum	after food
p.r.n.	pro re nata	when necessary
q.d.	quater in die	four times daily
q.h.	quatis horis	four hourly
stat	statim	at once
t.d.s.	ter die sumendum	three times daily
t.i.d.	ter in die	three times daily
Dx	gnosis (Gr)	diagnosis
Rx	recipe	take
Tx	trans(modern)	transplant

CATHETER CALCULATIONS

Description	Formula	Unit
Cardiac output (CO) (Fick, no shunt)	$$\frac{O_2 \text{ uptake (ml/min)}}{O_2 \text{ arterial content } (ml/\ell) - O_2 \text{ content MPA}}$$	ℓ/min [3–8]
Cardiac index (CI)	$$\frac{\text{Cardiac ouput } (\ell/\text{min})}{\text{Body surface area (m}^2)}$$	ℓ/min/m² [2.5–5]
Body surface area (BSA)	$(\text{height})^{0.725} (\text{weight})^{0.425} \times 71,84 \, (10^{-4})$	m²
Stroke Volume (SV)	$(CO/HR) \times 1000$	ml
Stroke Volume Index (SVI)	$$\frac{SV}{BSA}$$	
Systemic Vascular Resistance (SVR)	$$\frac{\text{Mean art. P} - \text{Mean RA P.}}{\text{Systemic blood flow } (\ell/\text{min})}$$	units [15–20]
Pulmonary vascular resistance (PVR)	$$\frac{\text{Mean PA P} - \text{Mean LAP (wedge)}}{\text{Pulmonary blood flow } (\ell/\text{min})}$$	units [1–1.5]

Note: Resistance = $\dfrac{\text{dynes/cm}^2}{\text{cm}^3/s}$ therefore 1 unit = 80 dynes s/cm⁵ and a pressure of 1 mm Hg is equal to a force of 1333 dynes/cm²

Pulmonary blood flow	$$\frac{\text{Oxygen uptake } (\ell/\text{min})}{\text{Pul. venous O}_2\text{content } (ml/\ell) - \text{PA O}_2 \text{ content}}$$	ℓ/min
Systemic blood flow	Same as cardiac output	ℓ/min
Left to right shunt (no bi-directional flow)	$$\frac{\text{Pumonary blood flow} - \text{Systemic blood flow} \times 100}{\text{Pulmonary blood flow}}$$	%
or	$$\frac{\% \text{ sat. pul. art.} - \% \text{ sat. mixed venous} \times 100}{\% \text{ sat. pul. vein} - \% \text{ sat. mixed venous}}$$	%
Right to left shunt	$$\frac{\text{Syst. blood flow} - \text{Pul. blood flow} \times 100}{\text{Systemic blood flow}}$$	%

Description	Formula	Unit
or	$$\frac{\% \text{ sat. pul. vein} - \% \text{ sat. aorta} \times 100}{\% \text{ sat. pul. vein} - \% \text{ mixed venous}}$$	%
Mixed venous saturation	$$\frac{2}{3} \text{ IVC sat.} + \frac{1}{3} \text{ SVC sat.}$$	%
Mitral valve area	$$\frac{\left(\dfrac{\text{CO (ml/min)}}{\text{Mean diast. filling time (seconds)} \times \text{HR}}\right)}{31 \times \sqrt{\text{Mean diastolic gradient}}}$$	cm² [5]
Aortic valve area	$$\frac{\left(\dfrac{\text{CO (ml/min)}}{\text{Mean syst. ejection time (seconds)} \times \text{HR}}\right)}{44.5 \times \sqrt{\text{Mean systolic gradient}}}$$	cm² [3]

HEART RATE/R-R INTERVAL CONVERSION TABLE

Rate (bpm)	Int (ms)	Rate (bpm)	Int (ms)	Rate (bpm)	Int (ms)
30	2000	78	769	170	353
35	1714	80	750	180	333
40	1500	82	732	190	316
45	1333	84	714	200	300
50	1200	86	698	220	273
52	1154	88	682	230	261
54	1111	90	667	240	250
56	1071	92	652	250	240
58	1034	94	638	260	231
60	1000	96	625	270	222
62	968	98	612	280	214
64	938	100	600	290	207
66	909	110	545	300	200
68	882	120	500	400	150
70	857	130	462	500	120
72	833	140	429	600	100
74	811	150	400		
76	789	160	375		

SYMBOLS AND MULTIPLES

Symbol	Meaning	Factor	
T	tera-	10^{12}	1 000 000 000 000
G	giga-	10^{9}	1 000 000 000
M	mega-	10^{6}	1 000 000
k	kilo-	10^{3}	1 000
h	hecto-	10^{2}	100
da	deca-	10^{1}	10
d	deci-	10^{-1}	0.1
c	centi-	10^{-2}	0.01
m	milli-	10^{-3}	0.001
μ	micro-	10^{-6}	0.000 001
n	nano-	10^{-9}	0.000 000 001
p	pica-	10^{-12}	0.000 000 000 001

THE GREEK ALPHABET

Greek character		Greek name	Transcription	
A	α	alpha	A	a
B	β	beta	B	b
Γ	γ	gamma	G	g
Δ	δ	delta	D	d
E	ε	epsilon	E	e
Z	ζ	zeta	Z	z
H	η	eta	Ē	ē
T	τ	theta	Th	th
E	ε	iota	E	e
K	κ	kappa	K	k
Λ	λ	lambda	L	l
M	μ	mu	M	m
N	ν	nu	N	n
Ξ	ξ	xi	X	x
O	o	omicron	Ŏ	ŏ
Π	π	pi	P	p
P	ρ	rho	R	r
Σ	σ	sigma	S	s

Greek character		Greek name	Transcription	
T	τ	tau	T	t
Y	υ	upsilon	Y	y
Φ	φ	phi	Ph	ph
X	χ	chi	Ch	ch
Ψ	ψ	psi	Ps	ps
Ω	ω	omega	$\bar{\text{O}}$	$\bar{\text{o}}$

Glossary

This GLOSSARY contains medical and technical words — and their meanings — that are commonly used in Cardiology and related fields.

A

ABC abb., Automatic Brightness Control (q.v.)

A MODE (Amplitude mode) An acoustic echocardiographic display in which time and amplitude are displayed along X and Y co-ordinates respectively.

ABERRANT VENTRICULAR CONDUCTION An abnormal intra-ventricular conduction originating above the ventricles.

ABLATION See under A-V Nodal Ablation or RF Ablation.

ABLATOR A radio frequency stimulator used for the ablation of conductive pathways and ectopic foci within the heart.

ABSOLUTE REFRACTORY PERIOD That period of the cardiac cycle during which electrical stimuli will not produce a propagated response.

ABSORPTION (Ultrasound) The portion of radiated acoustic energy that is absorbed and converted into heat as it propagates through body tissue.

AC abb., Alternating current. An electric current or voltage that alternates sinusoidally with time.

ACCELEROMETER A device used for the measurement of change in velocity and has an application in the pacemaker industry as a rate adaptive mechanism in VVIR pacing.

ACCESSORY PATHWAY An anatomically abnormal intra-cardiac conduction pathway between atria and ventricle allowing pre-excitation and/or re-entry, or circus rhythms. Its location is usually designated as either Anterior, Posterior, Right or left free wall.

ACOUSTIC IMPEDANCE (Z) The ratio of sound pressure to the particle velocity of acoustic radiation. A measure of the imped-ance of longitudinal signals as they pass through a dense medium. A product of the velocity and the density of the medium.

ACOUSTIC INTENSITY Acoustic power expressed in Watts per centimetre squared (W/cm²).

ACOUSTIC INTERFACE The tissue plane that exists between media of different acoustic impedances where some of the ultrasound waves are reflected and some refracted.

ACOUSTIC LENS That part of an ultrasound transducer that is used to refract the sound signals to a diverging beam or to a narrow focal zone. It is the component that determines the focal length of a transducer.

ACT abb., Activated Clotting Time

ACT MONITOR A device used to measure the adequacy of anticoagulation during cardio-pulmonary bypass surgery.

ACTION POTENTIAL The electrical variations generated by the cell membrane of a nerve or muscle cell after suitable stimulation.

ADAMS-STOKES SYNDROME see under Stokes-Adams syndrome.

ADAPTIVE RATE PACEMAKER A VVIR or DDD pacemaker, sometimes referred to as "rate modulated" or incorrectly as "rate responsive" that has the capability of changing its rate in response to metabolic or physical demand.

AFTERLOAD The forces resisting shortening of the myocardial fibres during contraction.

AFTERPOTENTIALS The dissipated energy through tissue after the delivery of a high energy pulse (not to be confused with Late Potentials, q.v.).

AGGLUTINATION The clumping of blood red cells due to antigen-antibody reactions or when blood temperature falls below 27 degrees centigrade.

AICD Automatic Implantable Cardioverter/Defibrillator. A device indicated for the treatment of VT or VF in patients who are at a high risk of sudden death.

AIDS abb., Acquired Immunodeficiency Syndrome.

AKINESIS Immobility (of the ventricular wall).

ALGIA A suffix meaning pain.

ALGORITHM The instructions and rules that are used by a computer to analyze data.

ALIASING A term used in pulsed Doppler echocardiography to describe the distortion that occurs whenever the velocity exceeds its maximum limit.

ALTERNANS (ELECTRICAL) An alternating electrical variation of the amplitude of the R waves caused by a reentry (q.v.).

AMBULATORY MONITORING Prolonged monitoring of physiological function by means of digital storage, frequency modulation on a magnetic tape or by direct radio transmission.

AMI abb., Acute Myocardial Infarction, q.v. Myocardial Infarction.

AMPERE Unit of electrical current. When one volt is presented across a resistance of one ohm, a current of one ampere flows.

AMPERE-HOUR The equivalent of one ampere flowing in a conductor for a period of one hour.

AMORPHOUS TISSUE A body tissue that does not allow the return of an echo pulse or beam of sufficient intensity for it to be measured.

AMPLIFIER A device whose output is a magnified function of its input.

AMPLITUDE 1) The height of an electrical pulse or DC level (either current or voltage), sometimes used in reference to calibration settings e.g. pressure manometry, flow measurements etc. 2) The output voltage and/or current emitted from a pacemaker.

AMPLITUDE MODULATION A transmission technique in which the signal of interest is superimposed upon a higher frequency "carrier" wave that will allow the carrier signal to be modified by the amplitude of the signal.

ANACROTIC NOTCH The interrupted or notched appearance of the ascending limb of the arterial pressure waveform.

ANAEMIA A quantitative or qualitative lack of or loss of blood.

ANALOG/ANALOGUE 1) Pertaining to electronic instrumentation in which data is presented by electrical signals of variable values of magnitude, e.g. the non-digital pure signals of a ventricular pressure waveform or electrocardiogram are both analog signals. 2) An organ or chemical compound having a similar function or pattern as another.

ANALOGUE/DIGITAL (A/D) CONVERTER An electronic circuit that will convert an analogue signal into a binary digital equivalent.

ANASTOMOSIS The surgically constructed connection between two vessels.

ANECHOIC The quality of a material that minimises or eliminates acoustic echos. It is used as a backing of a ultrasound transducer in order to eliminate reflections from its back surface.

ANGINA PECTORIS A recurring distressing pain of the chest that may extend from behind the sternum to the arms, neck and jaws caused by the insufficient supply of blood to a portion of the heart.

ANGIOGRAM An X-ray of an organ or blood vessels taken after the injection of radio opaque fluid.

ANGLE OF INCIDENCE The angle as related to the perpendicular (0 degrees) at which an ultrasound beam is directed towards an interface. The closer the angle is to the perpendicular, the greater will be the intensity of the returning echo.

ANNULAR ARRAY Referring to an echocardiographic transducer that has the elements arranged in concentric rings around a central point allowing gradable focussing.

ANODE 1) The positive element, pole, terminal or electrode of an electrical source 2) The rotating component of an X-ray tube from which photons are generated.

ANOMALOUS PULMONARY VENOUS DRAINAGE A partial or complete condition in which one or more of the four pulmonary veins enter the right atrium, vena cava or coronary sinus instead of the left atrium.

ANTECUBITAL FOSSA The part of the arm in front of the elbow where the forearm and upper arm join.

ANTEGRADE A forward motion, as in "antegrade flow" meaning a forward and normal direction of blood flow through the heart.

AS abb., Aortic Stenosis.

ASD abb., Atrial Septal Defect.

APEX The lower portion of the heart that is directly anterior, inferior and lateral.

ARC SCAN A technique of scanning echo signals that are transmitted through an arc whilst the beam is aimed at a fixed point.

ARP abb., Atrial Refractory Period. The period during which the atrium is unresponsive to an external applied signal. The total ARP (TARP) includes the P-R interval plus the post ventricular atrial refractory period. q.v. PVARP.

ARRAY Referring to (a) the physical arrangement of ultrasound generating elements. e.g. linear array when the elements are arranged in-line; Phased array; Annular; Rectangular; Hexagonal; etc. (b) an epicardial band or patch electrode used for the recording of electrograms during mapping of the excitation process. (c) the series of printing elements of a thermal array printer that create an image on thermoreactive paper.

ARREST (CARDIAC) A condition of either cardiac standstill or ventricular fibrillation that causes a fall of blood pressure and cardiac output. Cessation of normal electrical and/or mechanical function of the heart.

ARRHYTHMIA Any disruption or irregularity of the normal rate or rhythm of the heart.

ARTIFACT An aberration produced by some external influence or action. In reference to physiological recording, an abnormal extraneous signal e.g. as often seen on ECG recordings or an echocardiograph signal that has no anatomical correlation.

ARTIFICIAL HEART An prosthetic device manufactured to simulate the pumping action of the heart.

ARTIFICIAL LUNG A common name used for all types of blood oxygenators.

ASPIRIN A Salicylate discovered in 1763. Derived from the bark of the English Willow Tree (Salix Alba) and used today as Acetylsalicylic acid for the treatment of fever, pain and imflamation. It is also used as an anti-thrombotic agent.

ASYNERGY Relating to abnormal wall motion that produces a disordered time sequence of contraction during left ventricular systole.

ASYSTOLE Absence of mechanical activity of the heart in which the atria and ventricles (complete) or the ventricles do not contract, i.e. standstill, as a form of cardiac arrest.

ATHEROSCLEROSIS The slow pathological process of lipid accumulation, macrophage infiltration and muscle cell proliferation, commonly known as PLAQUE that lines the inner wall of an artery.

ATHERECTOMY Removal by mechanical means of atherosclerotic plaque from the intimal wall of an artery.

ATMOSPHERE A unit of pressure roughly equal to the mean pressure of the air at sea level under the standard acceleration due to gravity. 1 atm = 760 mm Hg = 10.5 N/m^2 = 10.6 dynes/cm^2 = 14.7 lbs/square inch = 1 Bar. To be more precise, standard atmospheric pressure is a pressure of 101,325 kilopascals, measured at sea level, at a temperature of 15 °C, at an air density of 1,225 kg/m3, and zero humidity.

ATRESIA A congenital absence or complete closure of an orifice or valve.

ATRIAL SEPTAL DEFECT (ASD) Non-closure of the atrial septum at birth, permitting blood to flow from one side of the heart to the other.

ATRIAL TRACKING A mode of pacing of the heart whereby pacemaker stimuli delivered to the ventricles are synchronised by sensed atrial activity. i.e. The VAT mode of operation of a DDD pacemaker. q.v. NBG code.

ATTENUATOR A portion of an electrical circuit that is designed to reduce the amplitude of a signal strength without distortion.

AUGMENTED LEADS Unipolar ECG leads designated aVR, aVL and aVF (augmented Vector Right...Left...Foot) are formed within the triangle of Einthoven (q.v.) by adjoining two adjacent apices of the triangle by resistors. This terminal point being one pole of the "lead" and the other being an electrode attached to either the right arm (aVR), the left arm (aVL) or the left leg (aVF).(F meaning foot)

AUTOMATIC BRIGHTNESS CONTROL (ABC) In reference to X-ray imaging, an electronic device that automatically maintains a constant light level of the output phosphor of an image intensifier. It has the effect of compensating for patient or tissue density during a radiographic exposure involving fluoroscopy or cine-angiography.

AUTOMATICITY The ability of the myocardial cell to spontaneously depolarise and to act as a substitute pacemaker which under certain circumstances may override the normal sinus pacemaker.

AUTO-REGULATION The process by which arteries dilate to maintain blood supply in response to an increase in demand, e.g. the dilatation of the coronary arteries in the presence of myocardial ischemia.

A-V DISSOCIATION A heart rhythm in which there is no relationship between contraction of the atria and the ventricles.

A-V INTERVAL Related to pacing, the period between an atrial (sense or pace) event and a paced ventricular event. See also P-R interval.

A-V NODAL ABLATION Therapeutic destruction of the atrio-ventricular node.

A-V BLOCK An abnormality of atrio-ventricular (A-V) conduction.

A-V JUNCTIONAL RHYTHM An abnormal heart rhythm caused by a pacemaker focus within the A-V junction.

A-V NODE The bundle of specialised conducting cells that regulate the conduction of the activation process from the atria to the ventricles.

A-VSD Also known as Endocardial Cushion Defect, this anomaly is a sub group of the ostium primum Atrial Septal Defect and is classified as either partial or complete, depending upon the involvement of the valves and ventricular septum.

A-V SEQUENTIAL PACEMAKER Any of the physiological pacemakers that allow sequential pacing of the heart.

AXIAL RESOLUTION The ability of an apparatus to distinguish two signals that are positioned along a common beam axis and in close proximity.

AXIS An imaginary line about which the heart rotates. It usually refers to the electrical axis of the P, QRS or T waves of the electrocardiogram as reflected on the triaxial reference system.

B

B MODE An acoustic echocardiograph display in which the intensity or brightness recorded on a cathode ray tube (CRT) is related to the intensity of the echo signal.

BACHMANN'S BUNDLE The anterior one of three specialised internodal tracts that are believed to conduct the atrial impulse from the right to the left atrium. The remaining two conduct exclusivly to the AV node.

BALANCING The adjustment of a baseline zero under conditions of zero output, e.g. of a pressure system, accomplished when the transducer is opened to atmosphere. q.v. ZEROING.

BANDING A palliative operation performed to decrease pulmonary blood flow in order to reduce pulmonary hypertension. It involves the placement of a restriction around the pulmonary artery and may be used in patients with transposition of the great arteries (TGA) or with ventricular septal defects.

BANDWIDTH The width of a frequency band that has an amplitude response that does not fall below 70.7 percent of its zero frequency value.

BARORECEPTORS Sensory nerve endings that are stimulated by changes in pressure. They are found in abundance in the arch of the aorta, the atria, the carotid arteries and in the walls of most blood vessels.

BERNOULLI EQUATION A complex equation relating to convective acceleration, flow acceleration and viscosity in a tube through which a liquid is flowing. It states that at any point in a tube the sum of the pressure energy, potential energy and kinetic energy is constant. In its simplified form, $P1 - P2 = 4V2$, it is used in echocardiography to estimate the pressure gradient across an obstruction, where $P1 - P2$ is the gradient in mmHg, and V is the measured peak velocity distal to the obstruction.

BICYCLE ERGOMETER A machine used to measure human work performance. The power (P) exerted $= 2.\pi.r.F.n$ where $\pi = 3.14$; r = the length of one pedal arm; F = the force applied to pedal and n = the number of revolutions.

BIGEMINY A regular ECG rhythm having complexes occurring in pairs of the same or two distinct morphologies followed by a pause, e.g. the repetition of a sinus beat followed by a VPB and a compensatory gap.

BINARY CODE The fundamental language of the computer. The system uses two numbers: 1 and 0 and relates to powers of 2 as compared to 10 in the decimal system.

BIPHASIC Containing a positive and a negative or an upward and a downward element.

BIPOLAR Having two poles or electrodes.

BIT (binary digit) The smallest computer information unit that forms the binary code. A unit of memory storage representing the 1 or 0 of binary language. 8 bits = 1 byte.

BLALOCK-TAUSSIG A palliative operation performed on patients with congenital heart disease with cyanosis (due to pulmonary stenosis or atresia with a right to left shunt at ventricular level) in order to increase pulmonary blood flow and subsequent oxygenation of arterial blood. It involves the anastomosis of the subclavian and pulmonary arteries.

BLALOCK-HANLON An operation performed on patients with transposition of the great arteries (TGA) to create an atrial septal defect in order to divert blood to the right side and better oxygenate the systemic circulation. It involves the surgical removal of the posterior septum.

BLANKING PERIOD The short time interval of ventricular refractoriness that is triggered by an atrial pacemaker stimulus during which the ventricular sensing circuit is inhibited. Its function is primarily designed to prevent crosstalk.

B.O.L. abb., Beginning Of Life. The indicators present when a pacemaker is manufactured that are used as a baseline from which all future indicators are compared.

BRADYCARDIA A slow heart rate, usually less than 60 bpm.

BROCKENBROUGH PROCEDURE A method of catheterisation of the left side of the heart. It involves the needle puncture of the intra-atrial septum through which a catheter may be introduced into the left atrium.

BRUIT An auscultatory sound caused by turbulence of blood flow across narrowed vessels or at high flow rates in normal vessels.

BUNDLE BRANCH One of the two branches of the bundle of His which descend through the intraventricular septum.

BURST PACING The delivery of multiple rapid electrical stimuli to one of the chambers of the heart. Often used to abort tachyarrhythmias.

BYPASS SURGERY A term used to describe the surgical procedure of diverting blood proximal to the narrowing of a vessel to a point distal.

BYTE A series of 8 bits giving 256 different combinations of binary numbers, each combination typically representing an alphanumeric character, special character or a computer control code. CABG abb., Coronary Artery Bypass Graft

C

CAD abb., Coronary Artery Disease.

CALCIFIED Referring to a deposit of calcium.

CALIBRATION The technique of checking and correcting inaccuracies of any analog or digital recording device. In reference to physiological pressure measurement it encompasses the static responses which include linearity, stability, drift and sensitivity.

CAPTURE The control of cardiac rhythm by an ectopic pacemaker or an applied electrical stimulus.

CARDIAC ARREST Cessation of ventricular contractility usually classified as either ventricular standstill or fibrillation.

CARDIAC INDEX The measurement of cardiac output related to the body surface area. Normal values 2.2 to 4.0 l/min/m2.

CARDIAC OUTPUT The amount of blood delivered through the systemic circulation per unit time commonly expressed in Litres per minute. The normal range is 4-7 L/minute.

CARDIAC TAMPONADE Compression of the heart due to the effusion of fluid into the pericardial sac.

CARDIOGENIC SHOCK A low cardiac output syndrome with hypotension accompanying severe heart failure that may occur after an acute myocardial infarction. The systolic blood pressure is usually less than 80 mmHg with a urine output of less than 20ml/hr.

CARDIOMEGALY Enlargement of the heart usually as a result of hypertrophy or dilatation.

CARDIOMYOPATHY Literally meaning disease of the heart muscle.

CARDIOPLEGIA Induced arrest of myocardial contraction performed during cardiac surgery by the injection of a cold solution into the coronary arteries (antegrade) or the coronary sinus (retrograde).

CARDIO-PULMONARY BYPASS A procedure that is used during open heart surgery in order to circumvent blood flow through the heart and lungs.

CARDIOTOMY RESERVIOR A container used during "bypass" surgery to collect blood from various suckers and vents.

CARDIO-VASCULAR Pertaining to the heart and blood vessels.

CARDIOVERSION The termination of a tachyarrhythmia by means of a synchronised direct current (DC) shock that is delivered to the chest wall during the depolarisation phase of the cardiac cycle.

CAROTID SINUS SYNDROME (CSS) The symptoms of baroreceptor hypersensitivity of the carotid sinus. Also known as Carotid Sinus Hypersensitivity (CSH).

CAST abb., Cardiac Arrhythmia Suppression Trial.

CATHETER A tube usually composed of a plastic material used for insertion into blood vessels through which blood may be withdrawn or various substances introduced. e.g. x-ray opaque media, optical dense dye stuff, drugs, fluids etc. When filled with saline it may be used as a pressure transporter when a transducer is attached to its proximal end.

CATHODE The negative pole, terminal or electrode of an electrical source, circuit or battery.

CATHODE RAY TUBE (CRT) The electron activated display screen of an oscilloscope monitor.

CAUDAL A topographical term used in reference to the view of the heart as seen from below.

CAUTERY The application of an agent that has the effect of destroying tissue. Q.v. Electrosurgical Unit.

CCD abb., Charged Coupled Digital. Referring to a digital camera used for X-ray imaging via a digital processor that produces a very high definition image.

CEPHALIC VEIN One of the two veins in the supraclavicular region commonly used for permanent pacemaker lead insertion.

CHD abb., Coronary Heart Disease. An occlusive disease of the coronary arteries, mainly caused by atherosclerotic deposits within the arterial lumen.

CHIP An integrated circuit. A miniscule piece of silicon crystal on which is etched a complete electrical, or "integrated" circuit. Used with other "chips" and discrete electronic components to provide a functional system.

CHRONOTROPIC Affecting time or rate.

CHRONOTROPIC INCOMPETENCE The inability of the heart to proportionally increase rate according to physical activity, stress and emotion.

CINEANGIOGRAM A cine film taken of the hearts action after the injection of an X-ray opaque dye into one of the chambers or vessels.

CMOS abb., Complementary Metal Oxide Semiconductors. A technology commonly used in the manufacture of integrated circuits that offers low power consumption. Commonly used in pacemaker manufacture.

COARCTATION A stricture of a large artery such as the aorta usually occurring at its arch below the origin of the left subclavian artery.

COLOUR FLOW IMAGING A type of pulsed wave Doppler that is used in echocardiography. It differs from conventional pulsed wave imaging in that Doppler shifted information is automatically obtained from multiple samples of a 2D scan.

COMMISSURE The line along the junction of two parts of a structure, e.g. between the leaflets of a heart valve.

COMMISSUROTOMY The surgical incision of the parts of a commissure to increase the size of the orifice. Mitral c. The separation of adherent leaflets of the mitral valve.

COMMITTED PACEMAKER A characteristic of some types of pacemakers that will always deliver an impulse regardless of the presence of atrial and/or ventricular depolarisations.

COMPETITION A competing rhythm in which the heart responds from two different foci such as found in bigeminal rhythm.

COMPLIANCE Having elastic properties. The opposite of stiffness.

CONCENTRIC LESION A narrowing of a vessel where plaque has formed in a symmetrical circumferential pattern.

CONDUCTIVITY The property of certain myocardial fibres to transmit electrical impulses.

CONSTANT CURRENT DEVICE A device that will emit a constant current irrespective, within limits, of the load applied across it.

CONSTANT VOLTAGE DEVICE A device that will deliver a constant voltage irrespective, within limits, of the load.

CONTRACTILITY A measure of the performance of left ventricular contraction that is related to the extent of myocardial fibre shortening and its velocity.

CONTRAST MEDIA A radiopaque iodine dye used for x-ray visualisation during angiography.

CORONARY Pertaining to the blood circulation of the heart which is supplied via two major vessels that branch from the aortic sinus known as the right and left coronary arteries respectively.

CORONARY ANGIOGRAM An x-ray of the heart during an injection of radio-opaque contrast media into the proximal coronary arteries. The technique involves the use of high resolution bi-plane x-ray equipment utilising closed circuit television, and an image intensifier operating in conjunction with a high speed cine camera.

CORONARY ANGIOGRAPHY A definitive diagnostic procedure for the evaluation of those patients suspected of having coronary artery disease.

COUNTERPULSATION The technique of increasing the diastolic pressure of the systemic circulation in order to enhance coronary blood flow.

COUPLING A heart rhythm where natural and ectopic beats alternate.

CRANIAL A view of the heart from the head.

CRITICAL DAMPING That amount of damping of an oscillatory system that forces attenuation of 50% at its natural frequency. It is the amount of damping that is just enough to prevent after-vibrations.

CROSSCLAMPING The action of clamping a blood vessel to avoid bleeding or to allow an operative procedure to be performed.

CROSSTALK The abnormal response to sense and/or record events from/to an adjacent channel, e.g 1) of a dual chamber pacemaker to sense a stimulus from an adjacent chamber such as the ventricular electrode sensing an atrial impulse causing inappropriate inhibition or retiming of the refractory period. 2) A high gain ECG signal that electrically interferes with the complexes on an adjacent channel. 3) Interference from one radio channel that is superimposed onto another.

CURRENT LIMITED DEVICE A device that maintains a constant current with the voltage varying proportionally with resistive load until the voltage reaches its upper available limit.

CYANOSIS The physical sign associated with an abnormal bluish appearance of the skin and mucous membranes, caused when the level of reduced haemoglobin within the capillary blood exceeds 5 grams, or one third, assuming the normal level of 15 gms %.

D

DAMPED NATURAL FREQUENCY The oscillatory frequency of a system on which damping has been imposed.

DAMPING Any means of dissipating the energy of an oscillatory system in order to reduce its amplitude.

DATABASE The organised files of information in a computer which may be retrieved, updated or merged.

DC abb., Direct current. An uni-directional electrical current of constant amplitude. e.g. the electrical current that flows from a battery through a fixed resistance.

DDD PACEMAKER A physiological pacemaker, that will allow the atria and ventricles to be sequentially paced and sensed and to operate in either a triggered or an inhibited mode of action;

DDI PACEMAKER A physiological pacemaker that will allow both atria and ventricles to be paced and sensed in an inhibited mode of action.

DEAD ZONE The area between the commencement of a transmitted ultrasound signal and its first identifiable echo.

DECIBEL The unit, abbreviated db, used to express the ratio between two amounts of power, either acoustic or electrical, existing at two points.

DEFIBRILLATOR An electrical device used for the termination of ventricular fibrillation and other tachyarrhythmias by means of a capacitor discharge direct current (DC) shock that is administered through the chest wall or directly across the heart.

DEPOLARISATION The sudden electrical response to a stimulus of an excitable nerve or muscle cell that causes the electrical potential to rise from a negative value to a slightly positive one during the initial phase of the action potential.

DEPTH The time duration between a transmitted and a received ultrasonic signal.

DEPTH OF FOCUS In echocardiography, the length of the focal zone.

DEXTROCARDIA A congenital embryological defect in which the heart is in an actual mirror image of its normal position, i.e. displaced to the right with inversion of the atrial and ventricular chambers.

DEXTROVERSION A congenital embryological defect in which the heart is displaced to the right as in dextrocardia, but with normal placement of the atria and ventricles.

DIAGONAL A branch of the left coronary artery.

DICROTIC NOTCH That part of the descending limb of the arterial waveform that troughs to form a "V". The notch is the minimal portion of the "V" wave and corresponds with the closure of the semilunar valve.

DIFFRACTION The distortion or scattering of a wave (ultrasound, light, electron) as it passes a geometrically disordered barrier, e.g. through a slit, around the edge of an object or a small body.

DIGITAL/ANALOGUE CONVERTER An electronic circuit that will convert a digital signal into a voltage output proportional to the incoming signal.

DIGITAL CARDIAC IMAGING (DCI) An X-ray technique that is similar to digital subtraction angiography, (q.v.), but is meant to obviate the motion artefacts that are present when angiographic studies of the heart are undertaken.

DIGITAL SUBTRACTION ANGIOGRAPHY (DSA) An X-ray technique that involves the use of an X-ray contrast agent that is injected into the blood vessels. Prior to injection of the opaque dye an X-ray image is made and stored in a computer. After injection a further image revealing the presence of the dye within the blood vessels is also stored. Subtraction by the computer of one image from the other produces a high resolution picture of the vessels.

DISTAL The farthest point. That part of a catheter, electrode, vessel, etc, that is distant to its point of origin.

DIVERGENCE In reference to ultrasound technology, the widening of the beam as a function of the distance from the source.

DOPPLER EFFECT The apparent change in frequency of sound, light or radio-frequency vibrations when the source and the observer are in relative motion to each other, i.e. the shortening of sound or radio waves when an object is moving toward the listener or receiver, and the lengthening of the waves when the object is moving away.

DOPPLER FREQUENCY The difference between the transmitted and received waves of an echo transducer that is proportional to the relative motion between the transducer and the interface.

DOPPLER SHIFT The difference between the emitted and reflected frequencies of the doppler pulse that gives information of the movement of the reflecting structure.

$$\text{Frequency shift} = \frac{2FV\cos\tau}{C}$$

where F is the emitted frequency, V is the velocity of the reflecting structure, cos (theta) is the cosine of the angle between the ultrasound beam and the direction of blood flow and C the velocity of sound within the body tissue (1560 m/s).

dP/dT A measure of contractility when preload and afterload are constant. A "change of pressure with respect to change in time". A physiological measurement rarely performed in a cath lab to evaluate the contractile velocity of the left ventricle.

DUAL CHAMBER PACEMAKER One of many types of artificial pacemakers that will allow depolarisation of the atria to occur prior to that of the ventricles.

DU BOIS NOMOGRAM A method used to calculate total body surface area from the known height and mass. q.v. Nomogram.

DVI PACEMAKER A physiological pacemaker that will allow both chambers to be paced after a committed atrial depolarisation.

DYNAMIC RESPONSE The fidelity with which a recording system will respond to dynamic events.

DYSRHYTHMIA An uncommon but more descriptive term of a disruption of rhythm. See also Arrhythmia.

E

EBSTEIN'S ANOMALY (1866) A congenital defect with a valvular insufficiency due to a downward displacement of the tricuspid valve into the right ventricle. The valve is so distorted that one or more of its cusps becomes attached to the ventricular wall.

ECCENTRIC LESION A narrowing or stenosis of a vessel where plaque is unequally distributed along its walls.

ECHOCARDIOGRAPHY A cardiac diagnostic technique utilising high frequency sound waves. These waves are transmitted and received via a hand held transducer placed in contact with the body at various sites, or windows, through which the ultrasound waves may readily enter.

ECTOPIC BEAT depolarisation of the myocardium that has originated from a pacemaker focus other than the sino-atrial node.

EDP abb., End Diastolic Pressure

EISENMENGER'S SYNDROME A congenital heart condition in which pulmonary hypertension is accompanied by a right to left shunt.

EJECTION FRACTION (EF) The percentage of the left ventricular end diastolic volume (LVEDV) that is ejected with each heart beat. It is the ratio of stroke volume to LVEDV. It is an important indicator of survival and a limited indicator of left ventricular function.

ELASTANCE In reference to transduction, is the total force exerted on a diaphragm to its equivalent displacement in the direction of the force. i.e. dP/dV or the volume elasticity coefficient.

ELECTROCARDIOGRAM The graphic presentation of the electrical activity of the heart.

ELECTROGRAM (EGM) The graphic recording of electrical activity.

ELECTROMAGNETIC INTERFERENCE (EMI) An artefactual interference superimposed on a physiological recording often originating from a high frequency source. e.g. diathermy, cautery, or any device that radiates electromagnetic frequencies.

ELECTROSURGICAL UNIT An electrical instrument that generates radio-frequency currents suitable for cauterising tissue.

ENDOTHELIUM The inner lining of the blood vessel.

EPI A prefix meaning 'on' or 'upon'. e.g. epidermis.

ESCAPE INTERVAL The period in milliseconds between paced or sensed activity and a subsequent delivered pacemaker stimulus. Atrial escape interval(AEI) is the period from the previous ventricular event to the delivered impulse to the atrium.

ESCAPE RHYTHM A rhythm that originates from an ectopic focus when the normal pacemaker fails to deliver a stimulus for one or more cycles. It may be either atrial or ventricular in origin.

EST Exercise Stress Test q.v. Exercise Tolerance Test

ETHYLENE OXIDE A flammable, sweet smelling, highly toxic colourless liquid that has a melting point of 10.7 degrees C. It is explosive when mixed with air at concentrations higher than 3 %. Commonly used for sterilization of materials that may not be subjected to high temperature or water saturation. When combined with an inert gas, its efficiency is dependent upon its concentration, humidity and temperature.

EXCHANGE WIRE A guide wire used during PTCA technique and introduced across a lesion for the purpose of interchanging a dilation catheter.

EXERCISE TOLERANCE TEST A study of exercise ability used to establish:- latent or overt heart disease; development of proficiency of an individual undergoing an exercise training programme; cardiovascular function. etc. The test may be MAXIMAL i.e. the individual is exercised to a level of intensity beyond which a further increase in the magnitude of work will not be accompanied by an increase in oxygen demand; or SUB-MAXIMAL i.e. when the workload is terminated at 85 % of the maximal age related heart rate.

EXIT BLOCK The condition of failed capture of the heart after the delivery of a pacemaker stimulus. It is usually due to an increase of stimulation threshold exceeding the output of the pacemaker.

EXTERNAL PACEMAKER A non-implantable artificial device that is used to stimulate the heart via an electrode or electrodes placed within the heart chambers.

EXTRACORPOREAL CIRCULATION The circulation produced by external means. e.g. by means of a heart-lung bypass machine where the venous return is by-passed through an artificial oxygenator and pumped back into the circulation.

EXTRASYSTOLE An ectopic beat coupled and dependent upon the preceding beat.

F

FALLOT'S TETRALOGY (1888) The most common of all the cyanotic congenital heart disorders comprising four main dysfunctions: pulmonary stenosis, ventricular septal defect, 'overriding of the aorta' and right ventricular enlargement.

FAR FIELD SENSING 1. Activity that is sensed by a pacemaker due to extracardiac signals. 2. The divergence of an ultrasound beam that is a function of distance from the source.

FASCICULAR BLOCK A classification of conduction blocks occurring within the intra-ventricular pathways.

FIBRILLATION An irregular uncoordinated rhythm of myocardial cells, which may involve the atria, ventricles or both. q.v. ventricular fibrillation.

FIBROSIS The creation of a stiff fibrous tissue within an organ, often caused by an inflammatory or hypoxic process.

FICK METHOD A method of determining cardiac output.

FIDELITY The faithfulness of reproduction of a recorded signal.

FILTER (1)That portion of an electrical circuit that controls the selective transmission of frequencies within the electro-magnetic and electro-acoustical range of vibrations. Filters are essential for the accurate recording of most physiological functions. (2) A device used in extracorporeal preparations for the filtering of blood.

FLOW-DIRECTED CATHETER A catheter that has a balloon situated at its distal end, which when inflated and the catheter advanced allows it to be directed with the flow of blood.

FLUTTER A rapid regular atrial or ventricular rhythm at a rate within the range 200-350 beats per minute.

FOCAL SPOT (of an x-ray tube) That portion of the anode of an x-ray tube that is bombarded by electrone emitted from the cathode.

FONTAN An operation performed to bypass the right ventricle in patients with tricuspid atresia or with single ventricle with pulmonary atresia/stenosis. It involves the anastomosis of the right atrium to the pulmonary artery.

FRANK LEADS (1956) An orthoganal system of electrocardiographic lead placement, commonly used when recording vector loops (vector-cardiography) and high resolution electrograms (late potentials).

FRANK-STARLING LAW A law that relates, within certain limits, the stretch of the myocardial fibres prior to contraction (preload), to the force of contraction.

FRENCH A measurement guage used to determine the diameter of a catheter or needle. 1 French size is equal to 0.3mm or 0.013 inches.

FREQUENCY (ELECTRICAL) The equivalent number of cycles/second expressed in Hertz (Hz). E.g. Power frequency : 50–60 Hz. Audible sound: 20–20,000 Hz. Radio frequency: 150 kHz – 1.0 MHz. Ultrasound: 1.0 MHz – 10 MHz. Microwave: 1000 MHz – 3000 MHz.

FREQUENCY RESPONSE The response of amplitude and phase as a function of frequency of an electrical or mechanical system.

FULGURATION The destruction of tissue by means of electrical current, e.g. during cauterisation and ablation techniques.

FUNDAMENTAL FREQUENCY The number of times a repetitive waveform occurs per unit time. All physiological pressure waveforms consist of a basic fundamental frequency on which is superimposed harmonics. (q.v.)

FUSION BEAT A beat arising from two simultaneous sources causing an aberrant spread of excitation and subsequent abnormal ECG complex.

G

GRID A plate of parallel strips of lead, separated by x-ray translucent material, that is normally positioned in front of the input phosphor of an image intensifier. Its purpose is to absorb and reduce radiation that is "scattered" from sources such as the patient, X-ray table and other ancillary pieces of equipment.

H

HAEMODYNAMICS The science of blood flows and energy within the vascular system.

HAEMOLYSIS The disruption of the red cell membrane causing the release of haemoglobin.

HAEMOSTASIS The cessation of a leakage from a punctured vessel.

HALF LIFE The time required for a substance to decay to half of its original value. e.g. A radioactive substance to lose half its radioactivity. An exponential function.

HARMONIC An oscillation of a periodically varying quantity having a frequency which is an integral multiple of the fundamental fresquency.

HEART FAILURE A clinical syndrome of effort intolerance due to a cardiac abnormality during whch the heart fails to adequately discharge its contents.

HEART MURMURS The vibrations caused by any condition that will affect either the flow or velocity of the blood within the heart or great vessels.

HEART RATE VARIABILITY (HRV) The measurement of the variability of the heart rate which is greater in the young and healthy and lesser in the aged and unhealthy. HRV is controlled by the autonomic nervous system and abnormal changes srongly correlate with arrhythmogenic complications and sudden death.

HEART SOUNDS The short duration sounds heard during auscultation of the heart by means of a stethoscope. Usually classified into (i) valve closure, (ii) valve opening, (iii)) ejection, (iv) mid systolic clicks, (v) ventricular filling (vi) and extra-cardiac sounds.

HEART TRANSPLANT See under TRANSPLANT

HEAT EXCHANGER A device sometimes used during bypass surgery in order to maintain blood temperature at a constant level.

HEMIBLOCK A blockage of electrical conduction of one of the two fascicles, known as the left anterior and left posterior branches respectively, that branch from the left bundle of His.

HERMETICITY The sealing property of a prosthetic device e.g. a pacemaker that insulates the interior from the outside environment.

HERTZ (Hz) The frequency measurement of 1 cycle per second.

HETEROTOPIC Pertaining to an abnormal anatomical position of a graft. e.g. heterotopic heart transplant.

HIS BUNDLE The bundle of conducting fibres that originate at the AV node and descend into the ventricles where it divides into its right and left branches.

HOLTER ELECTROCARDIOGRAPHY Sometimes referred to as Dynamic Ambulatory Monitoring. A biotelemetry system used for the recording and storage of the ambulatory ECG.

HUT Abb., Head Up Tilt Test. A test in which the patient is tilted up to an angle of 45 degrees after lying supine for a period of 30 minutes, during which time the ECG and Arterial BP are monitored. It is used to identify neuropathological (vasovagal) syncope.

HYPOKALEMIA An abnormally low concentration of potassium in the blood.

HYPOKINESIS A reduction of movement. e.g. The ventriculogram demonstrated inferior wall hypokinesis.

HYPERKALEMIA An abnormally high concentration of potassium in the blood.

HYPERKINESIS An increase of movement.

HYPOTHERMIA Low body temperature. Deep h; A body temperature below 20 degrees C, sometimes artifically produced during bypass surgery to cause cessation of the hearts activity.

HYSTERESIS Literally meaning 'to lag behind' or 'to resist change'. The pre-programmed condition of a cardiac pacemaker that will allow it to operate in two pacing intervals.

IABP abb., Intra-aortic Balloon Pump. q.v.

IDIOVENTRICULAR RHYTHM A conduction aberration when control of the heart is from a focus within the ventricular myocardium.

IMAGE INTENSIFIER An electronic tube used in conjunction with an X-ray chain that amplifies a faint image into a bright visible one.

IMPEDANCE Opposition to the flow of electric current within a circuit encompassing the effects of a resistance, capacitance and inductance.

IMPULSE A term used to describe an electrical discharge, e.g. from a pacemaker or an electrophysiological stimulator. Sometimes also known as a "spike".

INCOMPETENCE Lacking competency or efficiency. Usually used to describe the inability of a heart valve to perform its task causing regurgitation or back flow of blood from the chamber or vessel distal to the valve to the chamber proximal to it. Abbreviated 'I' with a prefix denoting a specific valve that is incompetent. e.g. MI,TI,AI,PI.

INFERIOR Situated under or low (opposite to Superior)

INFUNDIBULUM A funnel shape entry. Referred to the heart it is that part of the outflow tract of the right ventricle.

INFUSOR A device that is used for the administration, or infusion of intra circulatory fluids.

INHIBITION Related to Pacing — A mechanism that will cause a stimulus to be withheld after the sensing of a natural or abnormal depolarisation.

INOTROPE An substance or agent that will affect the force of myocardial contractility.

INPUT PHOSPHOR The illuminating or phosphorescent coated screen (cesium iodide) of an image intensifier tube where photons are converted from X-ray to light.

IN SITU To be in its original or natural situation.

INTRA-AORTIC BALLOON PUMP (IABP) A pneumatic pump device that is triggered by the ECG or arterial pressure waveform to cause an elongated balloon, positioned within the descending thoracic aorta, to inflate and deflate at specific times during the cardiac cycle.

INTRAMURAL Within the walls of a hollow organ or cavity.

INTRINSIC Inherent — Originating within.

INVESTIGATIONAL DEVICE An apparatus, instrument, electronic or mechanical device that is sold under the U.S. Food and Drug (FDA) investigational device exemption regulations.

IN VITRO An act performed outside the body.

IN VIVO An act performed inside the body.

ISCHEMIA The condition caused by a deficiency of blood in an organ.

ISCHEMIC HEART DISEASE An occlusive disease of the coronary arteries of sufficient degree to prevent the coronary circulation meeting the physiological demands of the heart.

ISOVOLUMETRIC PERIOD The period of early ventricular contraction when both the mitral and the aortic valves are closed and the ventricle is generating the force required to cause the aortic valve to open and overcome the diastolic pressure within the aorta.

J

JAMES FIBRES An accessory conduction pathway between the atrium and the lower part of the AV node.

J POINT The point usually accepted where the S wave of the electrocardiogram returns to its isoelectric line.

JOULE The unit of electrical energy. Power expressed in watts related to time in seconds. 1 joule = 1 watt per second or VIt.

JUDKINS A preformed stainless steel wire braided polyurethane catheter used specifically for coronary angiography.

JUNCTIONAL ECTOPIC TACHYCARDIA A rare arrhythmia that is peculiar to Paediatrics that does not readily respond to any form of medical treatment. It is believed to be caused by an abnormally situated His budle on the left septal surface of the ventricle.

JUNCTIONAL RHYTHM A rhythm originating within the A-V node or junctional fibres.

K

KENT FIBRES Abnormal bundles that form accessory pathways of conduction between the atrium and the ventricle that bypass the normal AV node.

KILOVOLT (kV) One thousand volts.

KILOWATT (kW) One thousand watts.

KILOWATT LOAD A term used to describe the amount of available power of an X-ray tube and its associated generator for a given time duration.

KUSSMAUL'S SIGN 1. distension of the jugular veins on inspiration seen in constrictive pericarditis and mediastinal tumour. 2. a parodoxical pulse. 3. convulsions and/or coma in gastric disease.

L

LAD abb., Left Anerior Descending branch of the left coronary artery.

LAMINAR FLOW The smooth flow of liquid or air, different layers of which move parallel at slightly varying rates, faster in the centre and slower at the periphery.

LAO abb., Left Anterior Oblique. An x-ray projection used during radiography useful for separating the ventricles and having the intra-ventricular septum in profile.

LAPLACE'S LAW A physical law that states that the tension generated in the wall of a spherical elastic thin walled chamber is the product of the pressure within the chamber multiplied by the radius of the chamber.

LASER An acronym which stands for Light Amplification by Stimulated Emmision of Radiation. A device that produces an extremely bright intensified light beam when high energy radiation is applied. It has many medical and surgical applications e.g. cardiology, gynaecology, orthopaedics, opthalmology, dermatology, neurology, etc. The light frequency produced by the device is dependent upon the type of gas employed e.g., carbon dioxide, xenon, argon or the crystals of Nd:YAG (neodymium coated yttrium-argon-garnet).

LASER RECANALISATION The technique of recanalising coronary arteries by means of laser technology.

LAT abb., Lateral or 'side-on'. In reference to radiography or angiography, a left lateral x-ray projection of the heart.

LATE POTENTIALS High frequency, low amplitude (HFLA) depolarisation signals that are present in the terminal portion of the QRS complex of some patients who have arrhythmias.

LEADS The insulated wire electrode used in a pacemaker system for the delivery or sensing of electrical signals to or from the heart.

LCX abb., Left Circumflex branch of the coronary artery.

LEFT BUNDLE BRANCH BLOCK (LBBB) A defect in conduction of the left branch of the bundle of His causing a delay in the depolarisation of the left ventricle.

LCA abb., Left Coronary Artery. The proximal segment of the coronary vessel originating at the sinus of valsalva at the base of the aorta.

LEFT VENTRICULAR ASSIST DEVICE A mechanical device that takes blood from the left atrium and pumps it into the aorta, allowing the left ventricle to be assisted and relieved of its workload.

LINEAR ARRAY A group of ultrasound transducers that are arranged in line and parallel to each other.

LITHIUM BATTERY The power source of most implantable cardiac pacemakers that use Lithium metal as the anode.

LOAD The resistance or impedance applied to an electrical circuit or source of energy.

LOWER RATE LIMIT The programmed rate of a pacemaker (DDD, DVI) at which pacing will occur during the absence of an intrinsic depolarisation.

LONG Q-T SYNDROME A congenital disorder that is accompanied by a high incidence of sudden death.

LOWN-GANONG-LEVINE SYNDROME A syndrome describing sinus rhythm with a short P-R interval without a delta wave believed to be caused by the presence of an atrio-fascicular connection.

LUMEN The open space within any tubular vessel or pipe.

LVEDP abb., Left Ventricular End Diastolic Pressure.

M

M MODE An echocardiographic mode of operation that displays the motion of intracardiac structures as echos of their depth related to time.

MAGNETIC RESONANCE IMAGING (MRI) An imaging technique that is often referred as Nuclear Magnetic Resonance (MNR). It relies on the physical principle that hydrogen atoms, when introduced within a magnetic field, are caused to align themselves. If an electrical frequency in the radio spectrum is aimed at these atoms they change the alignment of their nuclei. When the bombardment of the radio waves is stopped the nuclei realign and transmit small electrical signals which, because of the abundance of hydrogen atoms within the body, produces an extremely high resolution picture and, with the aid of computerised technology, body function can be evaluated. Unfortunately MRI equipment is costly mainly due to the expensive powerful electromagnets that are used. Patients with implantable pacemakers or other metallic objects within the body cannot be considered for imaging due to probable migration that would be caused by the magnetic field. The technique is becoming increasingly useful and important in the field of cardiology especially for the diagnoses of congenital malformations.

MAGNETIC RESPONSE A technique that reverts an implanted cardiac pacemaker to an asynchronous mode of operation (VOO or DOO) by the placement of a magnet over the area of the implanted unit.

MAGNETOCARDIOGRAPHY (MCG) A diagnostic technique that utilises the magnetic fields that are generated by the electrical forces of the hearts action.[82,83] The ECG, being a pattern of the electrical signals of the heart, generates magnetic fields that vary both in magnitude and direction. Although originally measured with inductance copper coils, these minute fields are today measured by means of highly sensitive instruments known as SQUIDS (q.v.) that are superconducting sensors that operate at minus 269 degrees C., i.e. the temperature of liquid helium. The successful non-invasive localization of accessory pathways in patients with WPW syndrome has been reported.[84]

MAHAIM FIBRES Abnormal bundles that form accessory pathways originating within the A-V node, proximal or distal bundle branches and end within one of the ventricles (usually the right).

MALLEABILITY The flexibility of a PTCA guidewire. Referring to its ease to shape or mould of the distal tip.

MANUBRIUM The upper portion of the sternum.

MARGINAL A branch of the circumflex artery of the heart.

MASTER'S TWO-STEP An exercise step test sometimes used for the measurement of human work.

MAXIMUM TRACKING RATE (MTR) A pacing term that refers to the programmed upper rate of an atrial tracking pacemaker (VDD or DDD) which is determined by the interval between paced ventricular complexes whilst a 1:1 AV synchrony is maintained.

MEAN The arithmetical average of a series of numbers.

MEAN PRESSURE The average pressure of a cardiac chamber or vessel. In the arterial system it usually approximates 1/3 of the systolic-diastolic difference added to the diastolic pressure.

MEDIAN The line dividing an asymmetrical distribution curve into two equal areas.

MEDIAN BASILIC VEIN A major superficial vein located in the antecubital fossa (q.v.).

MEDIASTINUM The central portion of the chest cavity bounded by the right and left pleura and the diaphragm.

MEMBRANE POTENTIAL The voltage existing during polarisation between the inside and outside of the resting cell membrane.

MEMORY The equivalent of one typed character measured in bytes.

MET Metabolic Equivalent that relates to the resting oxygen consumption of the body and is equal to 3.5 ml O2/kg/minute.

MI abb., Myocardial Infarction; Mitral Incompetence

MICROCOMPUTER A system that uses a microprocessor as its central processing unit.

MICROPROCESSOR That portion of a computer that controls all functions including logical and arithmetic operations.

MILLIAMPERE (mA) One thousandth part of an ampere.

MODE 1) The point of maximum frequency density or the most frequently occurring value within a series of numbers. 2) The method of operation of a device or action.

MODEM A device that will enable information to be telephonically transmitted between two or more remote locations.

MONOPHASIC ACTION POTENTIAL (MAP) The electrical impulse created from an instant change in voltage across the myocardial membrane.

MORBIDITY A diseased condition or state.

MORTALITY The death rate of any cause related to the total number in a group per unit time.

MS abb., Mitral Stenosis.

MUSTARD-SENNING An operation performed on patients with transposition of the great arteries (TGA).

MYOCARDIAL ELECTRODE A pacing electrode designed to be attached to the epicardial surface of the heart.

MYOCARDIAL INFARCTION A condition caused to myocardial tissue when acutely deprived of oxygenated blood, and if not immediately corrected, resulting in necrosis.

MYOCARDIAL OXYGEN CONSUMPTION The volume of O2 that is consumed by the heart and determined by the amount and type of activity the heart performs.

MYOPOTENTIALS The electrical signals emitted by muscle.

N

NATURAL FREQUENCY The frequency at which a mechanical or electrical system will oscillate when disturbed from its resting state.

NBG CODE A pacemaker identification code formulated by the North American Society of Pacing and Electrophysiology (NASPE) and the British Pacing and Electrophysiology Group (BPEG).

NECROSIS Related to the heart it is the irreversible myocardial damage caused by ischemia.

NOISE An aberration of a recorded waveform caused by some electrical event or mechanical vibration.

NOMINAL The optimum values at which any device is preset in order to permit normal operation.

NOMOGRAM A figure consisting of three or more lines each graduated for a different variable, that have a specific mathematical relationship.

NON-COMMITTED PACEMAKER Having no commitment. When related to pacing technology it is the mechanism whereby an intrinsic ventricular (or atrial) event will inhibit the delivery of a ventricular (or atrial) stimulus. See also under Committed Pacemaker.

NULL HYPOTHESIS Meaning there being no difference between two samples other than that of chance.

NYQUIST LIMIT A theoretical maximum frequency limit that can be accurately measured provided that the sampling rate, i.e the pulse repetition frequency (PRF) is at least twice the frequency being measured.

O

OESOPHAGEAL ULTRASOUND A technique of recording two dimensional (2D) images or doppler velocities by means of an ultrasound probe introduced into the oesophagus thereby providing an extra echo "window". q.v. TEE.

OHM'S LAW An electrical law expressing the relationship between voltage (V), current (I) and resistance R. V=IR

OM abb., Obtuse Marginal branch of the left circumflex artery.

OPERATING SYSTEM A software programme that will permit a computer and its peripherals to function.

OPTIMAL DAMPING The amount of damping that forces an oscillatory system to attenuate 22% at its natural frequency.

OPTICAL DENSITY The degree of blackness of a film image recorded by a densitometer.

ORTHOTOPIC Pertaining to a tissue transplant that has been grafted into its normal anatomical position.

OSMOSIS The movement of fluid from a region of lesser concentration to one of higher concentration when separated by a semipermiable membrane.

OUTPUT PHOSPHOR The second illuminating screen of an image intensifier that displays the light image to the cine and television cameras.

OVERDRIVE PACING The technique of pacing the heart at a rate greater than the patients intrinsic rhythm.

OVERSENSING In reference to pacing, it is the inhibition of a demand pacemaker by the presence of signals other than those which the pacemaker is designed to sense.

OVERSHOOT The initial portion of an underdamped pressure wave that is extended beyond the normal.

OXYGENATOR A device that allows oxygen saturation of blood cells. Membrane o. Blood and gas are separated by an artificial membrane through which gas exchange takes place by diffusion. Bubble o. Oxygen is "bubbled" or diffused through blood as a method of oxygenating and removing carbon dioxide.

P

P WAVE The portion of the electrocardiogram representing depolarisation of the atria.

PACEMAKER An electronic device that produces repetitive stimuli to the heart in order to depolarise myocardial tissue.

PACEMAKER MEDIATED TACHYCARDIA (PMT) A tachycardia caused by retrograde VA conduction during which the pacemaker (VDD or DDD) senses atrial depolarisation and in turn delivers a stimulus to the ventricle causing a ventricular depolarisation.

PACEMAKER SYNDROME The signs and symptoms associated with the loss of AV synchrony that is present to a lesser or greater degree in most patients who have VVI pacemakers implanted.

PARIETAL Pertaining to the structure or wall of a cavity.

PARTIAL PRESSURE The pressure or tension that a gas exerts in a mixture.

PATENT DUCTUS ARTERIOSUS The non-closure of the ductus arteriosus — that portion of the foetal circulation that communicates the pulmonary artery to the aorta — causing an enormous volume of blood to be diverted from the aorta to the lungs.

PATENT FORAMEN OVALAE A defect caused by a flap like tissue formed by the overlapping of the septum primum and the septum secundum within the atria through which foetal blood may flow from the right atrium to the left. At birth these flaps normally fuse together to form a closed atrial septum. Even when unfused the flap prevents left to right blood flow.

PATHWAYS The conductive fibres that communicate within the heart. They may be normal (A-V nodal) or abnormal e.g. atrioventricular (Kent), Atrio-nodal (James) and His-ventricular (Maheim).

PC (PERSONAL COMPUTER) An electronic machine that is able to memorise, sort, analyse and correlate data and produce selective information as required. It basically consists of a box in which is contained: (a) a disc drive, that reads information from a disc in the same way that a turntable plays records, (b) a micro-processor that performs all the logic and arithmetical functions, (c) two memories; a ROM (read only memory) that contains instructions for starting the computer and a RAM (random access memory) that contains instruction for the performance of a particular operator task. The task is entered from a disc or from a keyboard. The memory is measured in bytes (q.v.).

Connected to the computer is (a) a monitor, that displays the users typed information or instruction and the computers calculations, (b) a keyboard, that is used to send messages to the computer and (c) a printer that will produce paper copies of the contents shown on the monitor screen. The computer will house a 'hard' disc drive, and either accomodate a 'floppy' or a 'stiffy' disc drive'or both; all capable of storage of large quantities of data. It may also be connected to a modem — a device that will allow the computer to send and receive messages and data via a telephone line, or may be part of a LAN (local area network) system where data from many computers may be interlinked.

PCD abb., Pacing Cardiovertor Defibrillator. An implantable device for the treatment of tachyarrhythmias with anti-tachy pacing, cardioversion and defibrillation with back-up pacing facilities.

PD abb., Posterior Descending branch of the right coronary artery, although sometimes a branch of the circumflex in a left dominant condition.

PDA abb., 1) Posterior Descending branch of the right coronary artery. 2) Patent Ductus Arteriosus.

PE abb., Polyethylene. A plastic substance used in the manufacture of physiological balloons.

PERCUTANEOUS TRANSLUMINAL CORONARY ANGIOPLASTY (PTCA) The technique of dilating a restriction or stenosis within the proximal coronary arterial vasculature by means of inflation of a balloon located at the distal portion of a cardiac catheter.

PERCUTANEOUS TRANSLUMINAL MITRAL COMMISSUROTOMY (PTMC) The technique of separating fused commissures of the mitral valve by means of a catheter with an hour-glass shaped balloon at its distal tip.

PERFUSION Literally meaning "to pour through". Referring to the flow of blood through a vessel, organ or heart chamber measured in Litres or millilitres per minute.

PERFUSION CATHETER A PTCA catheter having a double lumen, one for inflation of the balloon and a second to permit perfusion through the coronary artery during the inflation period.

PERIPHERAL Superficial or close to the surface. On the periphery.

PERIPHERALS The components of a computer that are divorced from it. i.e. printers, disc drives etc. They are electrically connected via an internally located circuit card within the computer.

PET abb., q.v. Positron Emission Tomography.

PFO abb., Patent Foramen Ovalae.(q.v.)

PHASE RESPONSE The relationship between the phase of the output of an electrical or mechanical oscillatory system and the input.

PHLEBOSTATIC AXIS The level of the right atrium of the supine patient that approximates mid chest level.

PHYSIOLOGICAL PACING An A-V pacing modality that maintains atrio-ventricular synchrony by pacing the atria and ventricles sequentially; pacing the atria only (provided a normal A-V conduction is present) or pacing the ventricles after a sensed atrial depolarisation.

PI abb., Pulmonary Incompetence, Prothrombin Index.

PIEZO-ELECTRIC The feature of a substance to produce an electrical voltage when a pressure is applied to it.

PIGTAIL A catheter used for ventriculography whose distal end is shaped like a pigtail that allows it to retrogradely pass the aortic valve with ease.

POLARISATION The return of the cell membrane potential to its resting state after depolarisation.

POLYCYTHEMIA A condition where there is an excess of blood, that is expressed in relation to the haemoglobin or erythrocyte count.

POLYURETHANE A thermoplastic polymer used in some pacemaker leads as an insulating material.

POSITRON A nuclear particle having the same mass as an electron, but with a positive charge equal in magnitude to the negative charge of the electron.

POSITRON EMISSION TOMOGRAPHY (PET) A technique of blood flow imaging after the injection of a short half-life radioactive isotope e.g. N-13 Ammonia or Rubidium-82.

POTTS A palliative operation performed on patients with cyanotic congenital heart disease in which the descending aorta is anastomosed to the left pulmonary artery. Its purpose is to increase pulmonary blood flow and subsequent systemic oxygenation.

P-R INTERVAL The time interval of the electrocardiogram beginning at the onset of the P wave and ending at the onset of the Q wave. The normal range is 0.12 to 0.20 milliseconds and represents the velocity of conduction within the A-V node.

PRONE Lying face downwards. Opposite to supine.

PRELOAD Simply, the left ventricular volume at the end of diastole that determines the filling pressure (LVEDP) prior to ejection. It is the resting length or degree of stretch of the relaxed myofibrils. In any one ventricle of normal size and compliance either end diastolic volume (EDV) or end diastolic pressure (EDP) may be used as an indirect measure of preload.

PROPOGATION The spread of a waveform or excitation process through a medium.

PROSTHESIS An artificial substitute for a normal body part that is implanted within the body.

PROSTHETIC VALVE An artificial heart valve that is used to replace one that is diseased.

PROXIMAL The nearest point. The electrode of a bipolar pacemaker lead that is nearest to the point of connection. The point closest to the origin.

PS abb., Pulmonary Stenosis.

PTCA abb., Percutaneous Transluminal Coronary Angioplasty (q.v.).

PTMC abb., Percutaneous Transluminal Mitral Commissurotomy (q.v.).

PULMONARY BLOOD FLOW The flow of blood through the main pulmonary artery. It may be calculated by the formula:

$$\text{Pulmonary blood flow} = \frac{\text{Oxygen uptake}}{\text{Pulmonary venous O}_2 \text{ content} - \text{Pulmonary arterial O}_2 \text{ content}}$$

PULMONARY CAPILLARY WEDGE PRESSURE (PCWP) The hydrostatic pressure in the pulmonary circulation that is reflected in the pulmonary capillaries. It closely relates to the left atrial pressure and the left ventricular end diastolic pressure (LVEDP), in the absence of Mitral valve disease.

PULMONARY VASCULAR IMPEDANCE (PVI) The resistance against which the right ventricle must work in order to eject its stroke volume.

PULMONARY VASCULAR RESISTANCE (PVR) The resistance afforded by the pulmonary vessels to the pulmonary blood flow.

PULSE REPETITION FREQUENCY (PRF) The frequency or rate per second of the number of pulses transmitted/received to and from an ultrasound transducer measured in Hertz.

PULSE TRAIN A term that usually relates to echocardiographic Doppler colour flow techniques. It is the series of adjacent pulses that are transmitted sequentially in a given time i.e. the pulsed repetition frequency. For colour flow mapping the size of the pulse train is much greater than is used for M-mode and 2D imaging, since more energy is required for the transducer to detect the low-level blood cells. This is especially important when very small regurgitant jets are being mapped.

PULSED DOPPLER A sampling system of pulsed ultrasound that is triggered to transmit only after receiving returning echos from the previous emitted pulse.

PULSUS ALTERNANS A condition that is observed in patients with myocardial dysfunction where the pulses alternate in strength and amplitude in the presence of a regular ECG rhythm.

PUMP (BLOOD) An electrical device that is used during bypass surgery to maintain blood flow from and to the patient. Roller p. A valveless pump consisting of two rotating rollers that compress tubing in a circular raceway. Centrifical p. Having a rotating impeller that creates a pressure difference between its inlet and outlet.

PVARP abb., Post Ventricular Atrial Refractory Period. The fixed or programmed period immediately following a paced or sensed ventricular event when the atrial amplifier of a pacemaker is non-responsive to any ventricular stimuli or far field events.

PVC abb., Polyvinyl chloride. A plastic substance used in the manufacture of physiological balloons.

PYRO-ELECTRIC Crystalline materials that generate electrical current flow in response to applied heat.

PYROLYTIC CARBON A very hard black substance that is used in the manufacture of some heart valves and pacemaker electrodes. It is highly resistant to blood clot formation.

Q

QRS COMPLEX That portion of the Electrocardiogram that represents the sequential depolarisation of the ventricular septum, apex and base of the ventricles. It is measured from the first deflection of the Q wave from the baseline to the eventual return of the S wave to the baseline. Its width is normally less than 0.10 seconds.

Q-T INTERVAL The interval between the onset of the Q wave and the terminal portion of the T wave of the electrocardiogram. It bears an inverse exponential relationship to heart rate, i.e. as heart rate increases the Q-T interval decreases.

QUADRIGEMINY An arrhythmia in which there is a premature or any grouping of four beats followed by a pause.

R

RADIO-ACTIVITY The spontaneous disintegration of atomic nuclei which produces electro-magnetic or particle radiation.

RAMUS The artery located between the LAD and the CX often known as the 'intermedius artery'.

RANDOM ACCESS MEMORY(RAM) The memory of a computer that stores read and write information. It contains the instructions that the operator requires it to perform which is entered within the system via a keyboard.

RAO abb., Right Anterior Oblique. A radiological view used during radiography of the heart. Used to separate the atria from the ventricles and having the AV valves in profile.

RASHKIND The procedure used to create an atrial septal defect (septostomy) by either the use of a balloon or a blade.

RASTELLI An operation performed on patients that require continuation of blood supply from the right ventricle to the pulmonary artery, e.g. pulmonary atresia. It involves the suturing of an external conduit from the right ventricle to the pulmonary artery.

RATE MODULATION See Adaptive Rate Pacemaker

RATE RESPONSIVE See Adaptive Rate Pacemaker

RATE SMOOTHING The characteristic of some A-V sequential pacemakers that prevents the upper atrial or ventricular paced rate from deviating by more than a preprogrammed percentage from one cycle to the next.

RCA abb., Right Coronary Artery. Originating at the sinus of valsalva of the aorta, its major tributaries include the: sino-atrial nodal, conal, right ventricular, acute marginal, posterior descending, atrioventricular nodal and occasional left ventricular branches when there is dominance.

REENTRY Activation of excitable tissue caused by rapid and repetitive excitation via an abnormal pathway. To establish reentry three conditions are required: 1) A closed circuit of conduction, i.e. an antegrade and a retrograde conduit. 2) There must be a unidirectional block in one of these conduits, i.e. it must not permit conduction in both directions and 3) there must be a slow enough conduction that will allow the previously excited tissue to recover.

READ ONLY MEMORY (ROM) The instructions of a computer that are pre-programmed by the manufacturer for starting and loading. ROM memory cannot be lost.

REFRACTORY PERIOD The interval that follows any depolarisation in the cardiac cycle when no stimulus can cause another depolarisation to occur.

REPOLARISATION The changes that occur within the myocardial cell after depolarisation as sodium ions quickly diffuse from the cell and potassium ions enter.

RESISTANCE 1) The opposition to flow as caused by a restriction thereby impeding forward movement. 2) The opposition to current flow in an electrical circuit.

RESONANT FREQUENCY See "Natural Frequency"

RESTORATION CIRCUIT A pre-amplification circuit used in many ECG machines to offset the DC skin potential allowing a response of zero Hz.

RETROGRADE (V-A) CONDUCTION The condition in which a ventricular depolarisation is transmitted to the atria.

RF ABLATION The destruction of tissue by means of energy discharge from a radio frequency emmiting device.

RIGHT BUNDLE BRANCH BLOCK (RBBB) A defect of conduction of the right branch of the bundle of His causing a delayed depolarisation of the right ventricle.

RINGING A term used to describe the result of gross underdamping of an oscillatory system, usually seen as a series of oscillations following a high frequency signal.

RISK FACTORS Referring to coronary heart disease, those factors that increase the probability of acquiring the disease.

RMS abb., Root Mean Square. The measure of the average value of an alternating electrical current. It is 0.707 (square root of 2) of the peak voltage of a sinusoidal waveform and is equivalent to that power of a DC supply to a pure resistive circuit. Alternating voltages are measured on meters as RMS values, which means a voltage of 120 volts AC would have a peak voltage of 170 volts and a peak to peak voltage of 340 volts.

RR Abb., Riva-Rocci. An Italian Physician (1863-1937) who devised the mercury sphygmomanometer. The abbreviation is not often used in place of the more common letters BP (blood pressure).

S

SAGITTAL The anterior-posterior plane or section parallel to the median plane. MID-sagittal; A division through the midline into right and left portions. TRANSVERSE-s. A horizontal division through the midline into superior and inferior portions.

SAM abb., Systolic Anterior Motion. Referring to the anterior mitral valve leaflet, a consistent echocardiograph anomaly found in hypertrophic cardiomyopathy.

SCAN CONVERTER An analogue or digital device that converts one type of frequency into another. An example is used in ultrasound techniques where a converter receives data from the transducer and converts it to a frequency suitable to be displayed on a cathode ray tube monitor.

SCATTERED RADIATION X-radiation photons that are caused to be scattered or deflected from their original direction by the X-ray table, patient or other ancillary equipment and are not absorbed by the grid.

SCANHEAD The device that transmits ultrasound signals to the tissue under examination and receives the reflected echos.

SECOND DEGREE HEART BLOCK (2HB) Progressive lengthening of the P-R interval with intermittent dropped beats (Mobitz type 1 or Wenckebach block). A more progressive type occurs when the P-R interval is constant with cyclic dropped beats of 2:1, 3:1, 4:1 etc. frequency (Mobitz type 2). The lower portion of the AV node is usually responsible.

SELDINGER A technique in which a catheter is introduced by means of a guide wire.

SENSITIVITY 1) The ratio between the input and the output of any mechanical or electronic device. Most medically applied electronic amplifiers have a sensitivity control that permits the ratio (or amplification) to be changed. Sometimes referred to as a GAIN control. 2) Referring to the number of proven results of an investigatory test. The percentage of all patients with a disease in whom the test for that disease is true positive. E.g. If the sensitivity of an exercise stress test is 64%, 36% are false negatives.

SHOCK The condition of failure of the left ventricle to pump sufficient blood at an adequate pressure in order to perfuse the tissues and vital organs.

SHUNT An abnormal circulatory communication between vessels or heart chambers. They may be due to the failure of closure within the foetal circulation, congenital heart lesions or acquired as a result of trauma.

SICK SINUS SYNDROME (SSS) A term that refers to a collection of conduction abnormalities that mainly affect the normal function of the sino-atrial node (with possible involvement of the AV node) that are inappropriate to meet physiological requirements.

SIGNAL AVERAGING An electronic based technique that is used for averaging electrical signals that are regular and repetitive in character. It enables random stray signals commonly known as *noise* (q.v.) to be extracted from the original repeated signal, thus improving the signal to noise ratio.

SILENT painless, asymptomatic, occurring without any warning., as in SILENT ISCHEMIA.

SINO-ATRIAL NODE (SA NODE) The natural pacemaker of the heart. A narrow myocardial structure measuring, in the adult, approximately 3-4mm wide and 20 mm in length, located in the sulcus terminalis of the posterior aspect of the heart close to the junction of the Superior Vena Cava and the right atrium. It is the origin of the electrical discharges that escape to surrounding tissue of the right atrium.

SINUS ARREST A condition whereby the S-A node fails to discharge a stimulus for one or more cycles which usually allows junctional escape beats to occur.

SINUS BRADYCARDIA A physiological fall in sinus rate. Its cause may be due to an increase in vagal tone, an intrinsic depression of automaticity, a conduction block within the sino-atrial node or its surrounding tissues.

SINUS NODAL ARTERY The artery that supplies blood to the S-A node and surrounding areas. It arises from a branch of the RCA in approximately 55-65% and from the left CX in the remaining.

SINUS NODE RECOVERY TIME (SNRT) The time interval that occurs after the cessation of artificially pacing the atria (at a rate faster than the patients spontaneous rate) for the SA node to resume conduction.

SINUS OF VALSALVA That part of the aorta where the right and left coronary arteries originate. i.e. the bulbus origin of the aorta beyond the aortic valve.

SINUS RHYTHM The natural rhythm of the mammalian heart. Excitation originating specifically from the sino-atrial node which is sequentially transmitted to the myocardial tissue.

SINUS TACHYCARDIA An increase in heart rate above acceptable physiological levels (usually 100 bpm), the excitation of which originates from the S-A node. This condition may be caused by an increase in automaticity or by sympathetic overactivity.

SLEW RATE The rate of change of voltage divided by the time period in which that change occurs, expressed in mV/second. i.e. dV/dt.

SOMATIC TREMOR A baseline artefact superimposed upon an ECG caused by myopotentials generated beneath the recording electrodes.

SONE'S CATHETER A coronary catheter developed by Dr. Mason Sones.

SPACIAL VELOCITY PROFILE A map of the velocity distribution of a blood vessel across its diameter.

SPECIFICITY Statistically, the percentage of all persons without a disease in whom the test for that disease is truly negative. A conditional probability that a patient who does not have a disease will be correctly identified by a test.

SPECT abb., Single Photon Emission Tomography. A high contrast imaging technique used with the isotope Thallium-201 (q.v.) during exercise scintigraphy.

SQUAREWAVE The correct response of an oscillatory system that is damped sufficiently to avoid any under or overdeflections. It may be produced by a sudden change imposed on a pressure transducer when measuring the dynamic response of a monitoring system.

SQUIDS abb., Superconducting Quantum Interference Devices. Highly sensitive bio-sensors that operate at the temperature of liquid helium and have been used to measure the magnetic fields that are generated by the electrical forces of the heart.

STANDARD DEVIATION The measure of the length or range represented by the horizontal line of a Gaussian distribution curve. It indicates the dispersion of observations about the mean central point.

STRENGTH DURATION CURVE A plot describing the relationship between the amplitude and pulse width necessary to produce consistent capture of a heart chamber.

S-T SEGMENT That portion of the electrocardiogram that is measured from the point of return of the S wave to its baseline to the first upward or downward deflection of the T wave. Elevations or depressions of this portion of the ECG from the baseline are often indicative of ischaemic heart disease, pericarditis or other conditions of abnormality.

STENT An artificial blood vessel support used when replacing a valve or to improve suboptimal angioplasty results.

STAT With immediate effect — medical urgency.

STATIC RESPONSE The fidelity with which an oscillatory system will respond to stationary or slow moving inputs.

STOKES-ADAMS ATTACKS The symptoms associated with the conduction abnormality known as complete heart block. e.g. lightheadedness, dizziness and collapse characterised by sudden loss of consciousness with or without convulsions.

STRAIN GAUGE A measuring element usually embedded or bonded to an electrically insulated carrier substance. An electric current when passed through the element that is stretched or strained will produce a variation of current flow.

STROKE VOLUME That volume of blood ejected at each ventricular contraction.

SUPRAVENTRICULAR TACHYCARDIA A fast heart rate that originates from the S-A node or from any ectopic site above the ventricles.

SUPINE Lying face upwards. Opposite to prone,

SUPRA VENTRICULAR Arising from above the ventricle.

SVT abb., Supra-ventricular tachycardia. A tachycardia whose origin arises above the ventricles.

SYNCOPE A brief loss of consciousness due to a transient impairment of cerebral circulation. It is usually sudden in onset or may develop over a short period with symptoms of dizzyness and blurred vision accompanied with coldness of the extremities and sweating. Should the attack be prolonged a fit-like response may occur with convulsions that resemble those of epilepsy.

SYNDROME X A term used to describe the condition of angina pectoris associated with normal coronary vasculature. Positive exercise stress electrocardiograms are often recorded although normal angiograms may be demonstrated.

SYSTEMIC VASCULAR IMPEDANCE The resistance which the left ventricle must overcome in order to eject its stroke volume.

SYSTEMIC VASCULAR RESISTANCE The resistance offered by the systemic vessels to the mean aortic blood flow. It may be equated by subtracting the right atrial pressure from the mean arterial pressure and dividing by the cardiac output.

$$\frac{\text{Mean arterial pressure} - \text{Mean right atrial pressure}}{\text{Cardiac output in litres/min}}$$

The normal range is 12-18 units. (To obtain measurement in dynes/s/cm, multiply units by 80)

SYSTOLIC PRESSURE The highest pressure found in a cardiac chamber or arterial vessel during ventricular contraction.

T

T WAVE The waveform of the electrocardiogram representing repolarisation of the ventricles.

TACHYCARDIA An increase in heart rate in excess of 100 bpm

TAMPONADE Compression of the heart due to an increase in intra-pericardial pressure caused by blood or other fluid.

TCPC abb., Total Cavo-Pulmonary Connection. A development of the Fontan operation that bypasses the right atrium, conduiting the Vena Cava to the pulmonary artery.

TECHNETIUM PYROPHOSPHATE (Tc 99m) A radio-active isotope that is used for imaging of the heart of patients with acute myocardial infarction.

TEE abb., Trans Esophogeal (Oesophogeal) Echocardiography.

TELEMETRY The transmission of electrical signals or analog/digital data by means of radio frequency or telephone linkage. Information is relayed to a receiver and subsequently analysed.

TEMPORARY PACEMAKER See under External Pacemaker.

THALLIUM-201 An isotope used for exercise scintigraphy.

THERMAL DILUTION An indicator (temperature) technique of cardiac output measurement.

THERMISTOR A semi-conductor element that will measure temperature proportional to changes of its electrical resistance. Thermistors are used to indirectly measure blood flow (e.g. cardiac output

THIRD DEGREE HEART BLOCK or Complete Heart Block is a conduction defect in which the atrial activity bears no relationship to the ventricular activity and where the atrial rate exceeds the ventricular rate.

THRESHOLD 1. The value at which a stimulus will produce a sensation. 2. The minimum amount of electrical current or voltage that will result in a propagated response of myocardial contraction.

THROMBOLYSIS The action of dissolving, or lysing, of a blood clot by the injection of a lysing agent. e.g. streptokinase, urokinase, recombinant tissue plasminogen activator (tPA).

TILT TABLE TEST A diagnostic test used for identifying those patients who are susceptible to unexplained syncope. q.v. HUT.

TIME DECAY CONSTANT (TDC) The time required for an electrical quantity to rise to 63.2 per cent (1-1/e) or its final value to fall to 36.8 per cent of its initial value (1/e). where e = the exponential function 2.718. An important value used for the frequency response measurements of some older electrocardiograph recorders of which the TDC should be greater than 2 seconds.

TINES The projections located at the distal tip of some pacemaker electrodes designed to improve fixation of the electrode within the heart chamber.

TORSADES DE POINTES Literally "twisting of the points". The name given by Dessertenne (1966) to an arrhythmia that may be likened to a combination of ventricular fibrillation and ventricular tachycardia. During its alternating phases the complexes vary extensively in both amplitude and morphology and appear to change direction from one side of the iso-electric line to the other.

tPA abb., Tissue Plasminogen Activator. A thrombolytic agent that converts or activates plasminogen to plasmin by binding to fibrin. It is the resultant bound tPA-fibrin that converts the plasminogen to plasmin and dissolves the blood clot.

TRANSCUTANEOUS PACEMAKER An electronic device that discharges electrical impulses of constant short duration and manually variable voltage output, via two large electrode pads that are positioned on the anterior and posterior of the chest respectively. It is used in emergency during cardiac standstill or asystole.

TRANSDUCER A device that allows the transference of one form of energy into another.

TRANSIENT RESPONSE The relationship between the natural frequency of a manometric system and the damping imposed upon it.

TRANSPLANT (HEART) An operation involving the removal of the heart (organ) and its replacement with one taken from a donor.

TRANSPOSITION of the great arteries (TGA). A defect in which there is transposition of the great vessels leaving the heart, i.e. the origin of the aorta is above the morphologically right ventricle and the origin of the pulmonary artery is above the morphologically left ventricle.

TREADMILL A device used for the measurement of human work load consisting of a motor driven variable speed belt on which the patient may exercise.

TRIGEMINY An arrhythmia in which there is a continuous occurrence of an aberrant beat after two normal beats or any combination of three beats followed by a pause.

TRIGGERED A mechanism that will cause one event to be controlled by another. e.g. a DDD pacemaker that is caused to discharge a stimulus to the ventricle after a natural or aberrant atrial depolarisation is sensed.

TURBULENT FLOW The erratic pattern of blood flow created at and beyond a site of obstruction within a blood vessel or heart chamber.

U

U WAVE The sometimes present waveform that is seen after the T wave of the electrocardiogram.

UNDAMPED NATURAL FREQUENCY The frequency of an oscillatory system on which no damping has been imposed.

UPPER RATE LIMIT The maximum preset tracking rate of an AV sequential pacemaker.

V

V4R LEAD A Wilson chest ECG lead located over the 5th intercostal space, mid clavicular line on the right side of the chest.

V LEADS Wilson unipolar chest ECG leads designated V1..V6 and are formed within the triangle of Einthoven (q.v) by adjoining three apices of the triangle by electrical resistors being the true point of zero potential. The exploring electrodes are located at specific positions on the left anterior chest wall.

V-A INTERVAL The physiological time of retrograde conduction.

VALSALVA MANOEUVRE The act of a forceful expiration against a closed glottis that causes varying degrees of haemodynamic circulatory changes. Examples are straining at passing stool or during childbirth.

VALVULOPLASTY Literally the forming of a valve. The technique used in the catheterisation laboratory to open the adherent commissures of commonly, the mitral or aortic valves. q.v. Commissurotomy.

VAT A specific function of a pacemaker that will allow the ventricles to be paced, the atria to be sensed and to operate in a triggered mode of action.

VDD A specific function of a pacemaker that will allow it to pace the ventricle and sense both atrial and ventricles in either an inhibited or triggered mode. Often used with a single pass electrode that has its atrial contacts proximally situated to the ventricular distal pair.

VECTORCARDIOGRAM (VCG) An electrocardiographic display of the direction and magnitude (vector) of the instantaneous potentials of the heart during the complete cardiac cycle.

VELOCITY The rate of change of speed of a moving object, either accelerating or decelerating.

VENTRICULAR FIBRILLATION An unco-ordinated irregular rhythm emanating from resultant myocardial fibre excitations that produce chaotic and random movements of the musculature of the ventricles. This rhythm is fatal unless treated immediately by electrical shock therapy from a defibrillator or, for limited periods, CPR.

VENTRICULAR SEPTAL DEFECT A defect of the septum dividing the right and left ventricles.

VENTRICULAR TACHYCARDIA A regular heart rate of over 120 bpm that may be provoked by a single ectopic focus or by a reentry mechanism@located distal to the bifurcation of the His bundle.

VENTRICULOGRAPHY The technique of opacification of the ventricle with X-ray contrast medium during the procedure of cardiac catheterisation.

VENTRICULAR PREMATURE BEATS (VPB) Premature ventricular depolarisations that originate from an ectopic focus within the ventricular myocardium. They are characterised by wide and distorted QRS complexes and are often followed by a "compensatory pause" before the next conducted beat.

VISCERAL The inner lining of organs within the body cavity.

VOLT The unit of electrical pressure. 1 volt is maintained when a current of 1 ampere flows through a resistance of 1 ohm. 1 mV = 1 thousandth of a volt. 1 μV = 1 millionth of a volt

VSD abb., Ventricular Septal Defect.

VULNERABLE PERIOD The period of the cardiac cycle that corresponds to 20-40 milliseconds prior to the summit of the T wave. It is that part of the relative refractory period that is able to produce more than one response. Under certain circumstances this period of the cardiac cycle is considered to be hypersensitive to either artificial or ectopic produced stimuli.

VVI A mode of action of a pacemaker that will allow it to pace the ventricle, sense the ventricle and operate in an inhibited mode of action.

VVIR The NBG code (qv) of a Rate Modulated Pacemaker.

W

WATERSTON-COOLEY A palliative operation in which the ascending aorta and the right pulmonary artery are anastomosed.

WATT The unit of electrical power. The product of voltage and current.

WATT-HOUR The energy capacity of a battery or cell. It is the amount of electrical power that flows in 1 hour. Commonly known as a "unit".

WENCKEBACH PHENOMENON A usually transient incomplete heart block that occurs high within the A-V junction and is seen on the ECG as successive prolongation of the P-R interval until there is an isolated P wave with no related QRS.

WHIP The high frequency artefacts that are often superimposed on a recording of pulmonary arterial pressure. It is due to 'whipping' of the distal tip of the catheter within the artery.

WOLFF PARKINSON WHITE SYNDROME (WPW) An abnormal conduction defect that is characterised on the ECG by 'shortening' of the P-R interval. The P waves are normal followed by slurring of the upstroke of the QRS complex (known as the "delta wave"). The cause is due to the presence of an "accessory pathway" or conductive communication, between the atria and the ventricle that bypasses the normal activation process causing premature ventricular depolarisations, hence the shortened P-R interval.

WORD PROCESSOR An automatic computer programme used for writing, formatting and editing via a keyboard terminal.

X

XIPHISTERNUM or XIPHOID PROCESS The sword shaped cartilaginous tip of the sternum.

Z

ZEROING The process of correction of a zero level, required when calibrating a measuring instrument.

ZERO SHIFT The change of a zero baseline such as found during long term pressure recordings at high sensitivities. An ultrasound term used when the zero frequency baseline is adjusted in order to display a particular portion of the signal.

References

1. Marriot HJL et al, *Practical Electrocardiology*. Williams and Wilkins Co., Baltimore.
2. Rosenbaum MB. Types of Right Bundle Branch Blocks and their Clinical Significance. *J. Electrocardiology.* 1: 221 1968.
3. Hecht et al, Atrio-ventricular and Intra-ventricular conduction: Revised nomenclature. *Am. J. Cardiol.* 31: 232. 1973.
4. Tsai DS, Chen SA, Chang MS et al. A newly derived algorithm for the cardiographic localisation of Accessory Pathways, confirmed by radio-frequency ablation. *Abst. Vth Asian Pacific Symposium on Cardiac Pacing and Electrophysiology.* Aug. 1–4, 1993. *Pace* 16. #7, 1556. 1993.
5. *Special report: Instrumentation and practice standards for electrocardiograph monitoring in special care units. Task force of the Council on Clinical Cardiology.* Am. Heart Assoc, Oct 1988.
6. Slocum J et al. Computer detection of atrioventricular dissociation from surface ectrocardiograms during wide QRS complex tachycardias. *Circulation* 72: 1028, 1985.
7. Weber KT, et al. Identification of high risk subjects of acute myocardial infarction: derived from the Myocardial Research Unit cooperative study date bank. *Am J Cardiol* 41: 197, 1978.
8. Forrester JS, Diamond GA, Swan HJC. Correlative classification of clinical and haemodynamic function after acute myocardial infarction. *Am J Cardiol* 39: 137, 1977.
9. Packer M, Medina N, Yushak M. Haemodynamic changes mimicking a vasodilator drug response in the absence of drug therapy after right heart catheterisation in patients with chronic heart failure. *Circulation* 71: 761, 1985.
10. Morris AH. Editorial comment. *Chest* 94, 3: 455, 1988.
11. Gore JM et al. A community-wide assessment of the use of pulmonary artery catheters in patients with acute myocardial infarction. *Chest* 92, 4: 721, 1987.
12. Langer PH. *Circulation* 5: 249, 1952.
13. Kerwin AJ. Op cit 8: 98, 1953.
14. Gilford SR. Paper presented at AIEE-IRE Conference on Electrical Instrumentation in Nucleonics and Medicine, New York. Oct1949.
15. Masters AM. Test of myocardial function. *Am Heart J* 10: 495, 1935.

16. Rochimis P, Blackburn H. Exercise tests: A survey of procedures, safety and litigation of experience in approximately 170,000 tests. *JAMA* 217: 1061, 1971.

17. Bruce RA, Hornsten TR. Exercise testing in the evaluation of patients with ischemic heart disease. *Prog Cardiovasc Dis* 11: 371, 1969.

18. Ellestad MH. *Stress testing: Principles and practices*. 2nd ed. Philadelphia, F.A. Davis Co., 1980.

19. Patterson JA, Naughton J, Pietras RJ, Gunnar RM. Treadmill exercise in assessment of the functional capacity of patients with cardiac disease. *Am J Cardiol* 30: 757, 1972.

20. Robb GP, Marks HH. Evaluation of type and degree of change in post-exercise electrocardiogram in detecting coronary artery disease. *Proc Soc Exp Biol & Med* 103: 1960.

21. Mattingly TW. The post exercise electrocardiogram. Its value in the diagnosis of coronary artery disease. *Am J Cardiol* 9: 1962.

22. Diamond GE. The exercise test and prognosis of coronary artery disease. *Circulation* 24: 1967.

23. 23. Kattus AA. Exercise electrocardiography: recognition of the ischemic response, false positive and negative patterns. *Am J Cardiol* 33: 721, 1974.

24. Berbari EJ, Lazzara R, Samet BJ. Non-invasive technique for detection of electrical activity during the P-R segment. *Circulation* 48: 1005, 1973.

25. Flowers NC, Horan LG. His bundle and bundle branch recordings from the body surface. *Circulation* 48 (Suppl): IV–102, 1973.

26. Lazzara R et al. Electrocardiogram of His-Purkinje system in man. *Circulation* 48 (Suppl): IV–22, 1973.

27. Stopczyk MJ et al. Surface recording of electrical heart activity during the P-R segment in man by computer averaging technique. *Int Res Com Sys* (78–3) 1973.

28. Hishimoto Y, Swayama T. Non-Invasive recording of the His bundle potential in man. *Br Heart J* 37: 635, 1975.

29. Kienzle MG, Falcone RA, Simson MB. Alterations in the initial portion of the signal averaged QRS complex in acute myocardial infarction with ventricular tachycardia. *Am J Cardiol* 61: 99, 1988.

30. Gomes et al. A new noninvasive index to predict sustained ventricular tachycardia and sudden death in the first year of myocardial infarction: based on the signal averaged electrocardiogram, radionuclide ejection fraction and Holter monitoring. *J Am Coll Cardiology* 10: 349, 1987.

31. Mehra R, El-Sherif N. Signal averaging of electrocardiographic potentials: A review. Acupuncture & electrotherapeutics. *Res Int J* 7: 133, 1982.

32. Mahrer P, Young C, Magnusson P. Efficacy and safety of outpatient cardiac catheterisation. *Cath and Cardiovasc Diag* 13: 304, 1987.

33. Gruntzig A. Transluminal dilatation of the coronary artery stenosis. (Letter to Editor) *Lancet* 1; 263, 1978

34. Piller LW. *Manual of Cardiopulmonary Technology.* Chas C. Thomas Chicago Ill. & Staples Press London. 1964.

35. Norman J. An apparatus for accurate measurement of transmission delay time in catheter-manometer systems. *J. Soc. Cardiological Technicians of G.B.*, 3: 10, 1958.

36. Lilly JC. The electrical capacitance diaphragm manometer. *Rev. Scient. Inst.*, 13: 34, 1942.

37. Kern RE and Williams SB. Stress measurement by electrical means. *Elect. Eng.*, 65: 100, 1946.

38. Lambert EH and Wood EH. The use of resistance wire strain gauge to measure intra-arterial pressure. *Proc. Soc. Exp. Biol. and Med.*, 64: 186, 1947

39. Guyton AC. *Circulatory Physiology, Cardiac Output and its regulation.* Saunders, Philadelphia. 463, 1963

40. Kubicek WG. et al., Development and evaluation of an impedance cardiac output system. *Aerospace Med.* 37: 12, 1208, 1966

41. Starr L et al., Studies on the estimation of cardiac output in man and of abnormalities in cardiac function, from the hearts recoil and the blood impacts: the Ballistocardiogram. *Amer. J. Physiol.*, 127: 1, 1939.

42. Erlanger J and Hooker DR. An experimental study of blood pressure and of pulse pressure in man. *Johns Hopkins Hospital Rep.* 12: 145, 1904.

43. Remington JW et al., Validity of pulse contour method for calculating cardiac output in the dog, with notes on effect of various anaesthetics. *Aer. J. physiol.*, 159: 379, 1949.

44. Donal JS Jr. A convenient method for the determination of the approximate cardiac output in man. *J. Clin. Invest.*, 16: 879, 1937.

45. Kantrowitz A, et al. Mechanical intra-aortic cardiac assistance in cardiogenic shock: Haemodynamic effects. *Arch. Surg.* 97: 1000, 1968.

46. Weber KL, Janicki JS. Intra-aortic balloon counterpulsation: A review of physiological principles, clinical results and device safety. *Ann. Thorac. Surg.* 17 : 602, 1974.

47. Webb WR. Intra-aortic balloon pumping (Editorial) Ann. *Thorac. Surg.* 21: 521, 1976.

48. Holub DA et al. Changes in right ventricular function associated with intra-aortic balloon pumping in the cardiogenic shock patient. *Clin. Res.* 25: 553A, 1977.

49. Mason DT et al. Diagnosis and management of myocardial infarction shock. In Elliot RS et al. *Cardiac Emergencies*. 2nd Ed. Mount Kisco, N.Y., Futura. 1982.

50. *Lithium based batteries for pacemaker applications: A technical overview*. Mosharrafa M, Technical note No. 10, Cardiac Pacemakers Inc., St. Paul, Min. 1976.

51. Berstein et al, The NASPE/BPEG generic code for antibradyarrhythmia and adaptive-rate pacing and anti-tachyarrhythmia devices. *Pace*, 10: 1, 1987.

52. Bredakis JJ and Stirbys PP. A suggested code for permanent pacing leads. *Pace*, 8: 1, 1985.

53. Kaul U, Grigg L. Cardiac pacing in sino-atrial bradycardias. *Clin Progress*. 3 (2): 130, 1985.

54. Levine PA, Mace RC. In 'Pacing Therapy', Futura Pub. Coy. Inc. New York. 1983.

55. Wirtzfeld A, Schmidt C, Himmler C, Stangl K. Physiological pacing: Present status and future developments. *Pace*, 10: 48. 1987.

56. Furman S. *4th European Symposium on Cardiac Pacing*. Stockholm 1989.

57. Lown B, Ameresingham R, Newman J. New method for terminating cardiac arrhythmias. *JAMA* 182: 548, 1962.

58. Provost JL. Battelli F. La mort par les decharges electriques. *J. de physiol at de path. gen.* 1: 399, 427 1899.

59. Scheinman MM, Morady F, Hess DS, et al: Catheter induced ablation of the atrio-ventricular junction to control refractory supra-ventricular arrhythmias. *JAMA.*, 248: 851, 1982.

60. Holt P, Boyd EGCA. Endocardial ablation: The background to its use in ventricular tachycardia. *Br. Heart J.* 51: 687. 1984.

61. Fisher JD, Kim SG, Matos JA et al. Complications of catheter ablation of tachyarrhythmias: Occurrence, protection and prevention. *Clin. Prog. Electrophysiol. and Pacing.* 3: 292, 1985.

62. Huang SKS et al. Radiofrequency catheter ablation of the atrioventricular junction for refractory supraventricular tachycardia (abstract). *Circulation* 78 (Suppl II): II-156, 1988.

63. Lavergne TL et al. Transcatheter radiofrequency modification of atrioventricular conduction for /refractory supraventricular tachycardia (abstract). *Circulation* 78 (Suppl II): II-305, 1988.

64. Jackman WM et al. Catheter ablation of the atrioventricular junction using radiofrequency current in 17 patients. *Circulation* 83: No. 5, 1562, 1991.

65. Editorial. Catheter ablation for supraventricular tachycardia. *Ed. N Engl J Med* 324: 1661, 1991.

66. Calkins MD et al. Diagnosis and cure of WPW syndrome or paroxysmal supraventricular tachycardias during a single electrophysiology test. *N Engl J Med* 324: 1612, 1991.

67. Jackman WM et al. Catheter ablation of accessory atrioventricular pathways (Wolff-Parkinson-White syndrome) by radio-frequency current. *N Engl J Med* 324: 1606, 1991.

68. Lee MA et al. Catheter modification of the atrioventricular junction with radio frequency energy for control of atrioventricular nodal reentry tachycardia. *Circulation* 83: 827, 1991.

69. Langberg JJ et al. Radiofrequency catheter ablation: The effect of electrode size on lesion volume in vivo. *Pace* 13: 1242, 1990.

70. Hatle L, Angelsen B. *Doppler Ultrasound in Cardiology*, 2nd Ed., Lea & Febiger, Philadelphia. 1985.

71. Weyman. Arthur. *Principles and Practices of Echocardiography*. 2nd Edition. Lea and Febiger. Philadelphia. 1994.

72. Wilde P. *Doppler Echocardiography: An illustrated clinical guide*. Churchill Livingstone, Edinburgh.1989.

73. Amon, Fatal shock from a cardiac monitor. *The Lancet*, 1: 872. 1960.

74. Dalziel CF, *The effects of electric shock on man*. U.S. Atomic Energy Commission. 1956.

75. Dalziel CF, Dangerous electric currents. *AIEE trans. Elect. Engineering*, 65: 579, 1946.

76. Daziel CF & Lee WR, Lethal electric currents. *IEEE Spectrum*, 44, February 1969.

77. Burchell HB, Electrocution hazards in the hospital or laboratory. *Circulation*, 27: 1015, 1963.

78. Starmer CF at al, Hazards of electric shock in cardiology. *Amer. J. Cardio.*, 14: 537 1964.

79. Whalen RE, Starmer CF, Electric shock hazards in clinical cardiology. *Modern Concepts in Cardiovascular Disease*, 36: No. 2 Feb. 1967.

80. Freiberger H, The electrical resistance of the human body to DC and AC currents. *Elektrizitatswirtschaft*. Berlin. 5th September 1933.

81. Dalziel CF and Lee WR, Re-evaluation of lethal electric currents. IEEE Trans. Industry and General Applications. *IGA*-4: 467, 1968.

82. Baule GM, Theory of magnetic detection of the hearts electrical activity. *J.Appl. Phys.* 36: 2006, 1965.

83. Gudden F, Hoenig H et al. A multi-channel system for use in biomagnetic diagnoses in neurology and cardology. *Electromedica*. 57: No.1. 1989.

84. Moshage W. et al. Magnetocardiography: non-invasive localisation of accessory pathways in patients with Wolff-Parkinson-White Syndrome. *Electromedica*. 57: No.4, 122. 1989.

Index